Career Planning for Doctors

Career Planning for Doctors

An Evidence-Based Guide

Caroline Elton
Associate Professor of Medical Education and Careers Lead,
Norwich Medical School, Norwich, UK

Naomi Elton
Systemic Therapist, The Family Treatment Service,
London, UK
Retired Consultant Psychiatrist, Cambridge, UK

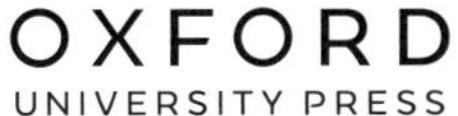

OXFORD
UNIVERSITY PRESS

Great Clarendon Street, Oxford, OX2 6DP,
United Kingdom

Oxford University Press is a department of the University of Oxford.
It furthers the University's objective of excellence in research, scholarship,
and education by publishing worldwide. Oxford is a registered trade mark of
Oxford University Press in the UK and in certain other countries.

Published in the United States of America by Oxford University Press
198 Madison Avenue, New York, NY 10016, United States of America.

British Library Cataloguing in Publication Data
Data available

Library of Congress Control Number: 2025933989

ISBN 978–0–19–888487–3

DOI: 10.1093/med/9780198884873.001.0001

Printed in the UK by
Bell & Bain Ltd., Glasgow

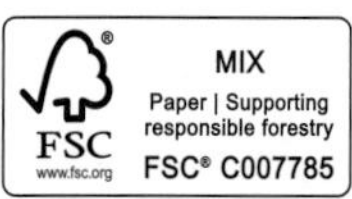

Foreword

In my second year at medical school in India, decades ago, I was cycling downhill to the hostel having just come out of the dissection room and attended physiology lectures in the morning. I was mulling over that morning's experiences. I thought to myself that we all have roughly similar anatomy and physiology and wondered what makes each of us different? That was the point when I got interested in psychiatry. Everyone I talked to subsequently told me that I must be crazy if I wanted to do psychiatry. Having listened to their objections, I did work in surgical and medical specialities before finding my home in psychiatry.

Why do people want to be doctors? Often, it is a personal choice with a commitment to help those who need help and support. Others may want to help humanity through medical research or combine their interests in both teaching and medicine. These decisions may follow a previous minor or major experience whereas others may choose medicine because of parental pressure, ambition or academic achievement. Once an individual has been through 4 or 5 years of arduous learning and training, they begin to feel that the end is in sight. However, often that is the beginning of choosing a specialty.

Medicine is a vocation and a profession. It is an art and a science. Traditionally medical specialties have often been divided into arts and craft specialties. However, as medicine becomes more technical, the overlap between art and craft becomes less clear. Medical students have often complained to me that they went into medicine to serve suffering humanity and not to be technicians. However, it is crucial to acknowledge that technology can be a very helpful tool for assisting the clinician to provide the right interventions and improve outcomes.

In many countries, parents of doctors push their children to go into the same specialty they are themselves working in, so that they may be able to hand over their clinics and services to their children—who may thus have limited choice. In other settings, specialty choice may be impulsively or carefully selected. Some students 'fall' into a specialty for practical reasons. Some specialty options are relatively easy to get into whereas others may be more difficult to attain. Many students have gone into medicine with a clear idea of what they wanted to do; in which specialty they wanted to work. A proportion of students may have no idea about their choice of specialty when they enter medical school. Others may start training in one specialty but switch to another. These choices are individual and will be affected very strongly by the availability of training posts.

Many doctors struggle to choose a specialty, then worry about whether they have made the right decision. These doubts can affect their progress and functioning as well as their retention in the field. Increasingly doctors may choose to take time off travelling or spend time abroad for training or working in a different healthcare system.

In choosing the specialty that one may want to work in, it is helpful to be aware of one's own skills and strengths as well as one's weaknesses. Even though it may appear that once a doctor has chosen a specialty it is for life, within each specialty job portfolios can be created, the components of which can be changed. In many specialties, it is possible and indeed helpful to move from one type of clinical service to another, add teaching, policy development, or medical politics to stay fresh.

There are alternative and unusual options available. I was surprised, when I met a doctor who had graduated and decided to give up medicine and become a pianist instead. Another colleague who went into psychiatry while remaining a concert-level pianist, now gives talks about the mental health of various composers and their mental states when they composed certain pieces, demonstrating these through playing.

The authors Caroline Elton and Naomi Elton (not related) are well-placed to write this volume. Both have been involved in educating and supporting trainees and medical students. Not only do the authors set the scene in an easy-to-follow manner, but each chapter is also full of practical advice which would help both students and educators. Each chapter illustrates theoretical points with various helpful exercises with an indication of the rough time each exercise may take which allows suitable preparation. They highlight work values which need a degree of prioritization. Creating a list of one's own likes and dislikes can help any individual to reach an informed decision. This will include an emphasis on work-life balance.

The practical advice they offer is that students need to *plan* for specialty selection. This planning should be done in stages. They advise that medical students can benefit from making a longlist of specialties and then a shortlist. Additional factors such as whether they wish to follow research, or academic careers must be taken into account. There will be questions at each stage which need addressing. This is where informed decision-making comes into play. As the authors highlight, students can explore these in detail before making up their mind. These include discussions and support from their supervisors and tutors. Part-time attachments, special interest, or taster days can expand one's exposure to a range of specialties. The authors recommend that students attend conferences, public lectures and talks to gain different perspectives which could be extremely helpful in reaching a decision. The students should also get involved in various research opportunities. They need to gather information from multiple sources. All these experiences can help them make the right decision. The authors encourage the students to have a back-up option too. They recommend that students think 5 to 10 years ahead, taking personal and professional factors into account before making their choice of specialty. In addition, they provide advice on getting the priorities right and how to submit applications. They suggest that students need to be aware of optimism bias as well as competition ratios and the availability of vacancies.

Global movement of doctors from high-income countries to other high-income countries and from low and middle-income countries to high-income countries plays a role in finding short and long-term training posts. This may contribute to stress and burnout and the authors offer a very helpful guide to resilience and well-being. Career success and satisfaction are important but should not be the only outcome but one among many.

The authors have considered more vulnerable groups such as international medical graduates and refugee doctors, for which we must be grateful. The needs and experiences of these groups will be different. As the authors recommend, courage and patience, learning from failure and from success are part of personal growth.

The book is full of sound, practical, and helpful advice. The authors deserve our congratulations and thanks for putting together an advice manual that should be a compulsory read for medical students, doctors at all levels of training as well as educational and clinical supervisors, and mentors.

Dinesh Bhugra, CBE

MA, MSc, MBBS, DSc (Hon), PhD, FRCP, FRCPE, FRCPsych, FFPHM, FRCPsych(Hon), FHKCPsych(Hon), FACPsych(Hon), FAMS(Singapore), FKCL, MPhil, LMSSA, FAcadME, FRSA, DIFAPA

Professor Emeritus, Mental Health & Cultural Diversity, IoPPN, Kings College London

President, Royal College of Psychiatrists (2008–2011)

President, World Psychiatric Association (2014–2017)

President, British Medical Association (2018–2019)

President, Mental Health Foundation (2014–2020)

Acknowledgements

Our work with very many doctors and medical students has allowed us to write this book. Some have allowed us to share their experience, appropriately anonymized, directly, while others contributed indirectly by adding to the tacit knowledge that we have shared in this book. All the doctors and students with whom we have worked have encouraged our writing, urging us to put something out there for the benefit of colleagues facing career decisions, sometimes with minimal support.

We want to acknowledge the role models each of us has had over the course of our own careers: those who listened, problem-solved, supported, and asked difficult questions, sometimes challenging the 'received wisdom' as to how things needed to be done. Doctors who were crucial to Naomi's development included the late Prof Bob Cawley, Caroline Garland, Dr Jonathan Dare, Dr Alan Cooklin, and Dr Margaret Murphy. As stand-out role models, these doctors informed this book, in some cases, many decades ago. Caroline would like to acknowledge the late Professor Kath Green, Professor Dane Goodsman, Dr Andrew Long, Dr Camilla Kingdon, and Dr Maggie Bunting—all of whom nurtured her career as a psychologist working in medical education.

We want to thank our families—Andrew, Jonathan, Tim, Jonty, and Nat in particular for their encouragement, foundation-doctor perspective, help with figures, critique, and manuscript reading. We also want to thank OUP for publishing this book. We had intended to conclude our acknowledgements by expressing our gratitude to our talented illustrator Dr Paula Heister. Not only did Paula create the illustrations, but she also agreed to feature in a case study. But during the publication period, Paula was diagnosed with an aggressive brain tumour and she died just two months later. This book is dedicated to her.

Contents

About the authors

Caroline Elton is an occupational psychologist who specializes in medical career coaching. Following her first degree at Oxford University and postgraduate scholarship to the University of Pennsylvania, she trained as an inner-city secondary school teacher. After a number of years she changed career direction, undertaking a PhD in the Department of Academic Psychiatry at the Middlesex Hospital in London. Having switched careers herself, she became interested in the psychology of work, and later trained as both an occupational and counselling psychologist. For over 25 years Caroline has held a number of senior roles in medical education. In 2008 she set up and then ran the London Deanery Careers Unit providing a careers support service for all trainees working across the capital. This experience formed the basis of her book *Also Human: The Inner Lives of Doctors*, published in 2018 by Penguin Random House. Currently Caroline is Associate Professor in Medical Education and Career Lead at Norwich Medical School.

Naomi Elton is a doctors' career coach and systemic therapist. Naomi's undergraduate medical training was at The Middlesex Hospital Medical School, graduating from UCLH. She later trained in psychiatry at the Maudsley Hospital and in child and adolescent psychiatry (CAMHS) at Great Ormond St Hospital, London. As a CAMHS consultant, she worked in Cambridge, Essex, Huntingdon, and Peterborough, her practice always being informed by systemic thinking. To work systemically is to be continually curious about our relationships and ourselves—how things join up. It's also about turning the microscope on oneself. Mid-career, Naomi studied for a master's degree in occupational psychology at Birkbeck, University of London. She went on to lead the children's community services in her NHS organization for several years, modernizing services, and mitigating the impact of austerity on children's services and staff. Naomi then took the plunge to work independently as a coach and a systemic therapist.

Caroline and Naomi share the same surname, and the same approach to career coaching—but are not in fact related.

About the illustrator Dr Paula Heister, 1984–2025

Paula was a doctor, scientist, author, and illustrator. She gained a D.Phil in Pharmacology from the University of Oxford and completed her medical training at Imperial College London. But Paula was also passionate about art. Despite having no formal art training, she was accepted onto an M.A. course in Children's Book Illustration at the Cambridge School of Art. After graduating, Paula combined her career as an artist and author with teaching medicine at Downing College, Cambridge.

In 2025, Paula was awarded a fellowship at the Harvard Radcliffe Institute. She aimed to write and illustrate a picture book for school age children on the science and practicalities surrounding death. In a cruel irony, Paula herself became ill and died before she could start her fellowship.

Caroline and Naomi are honoured to be able to showcase Paula's illustrations in this book.

How to use this book

This is a book for all medical students and doctors facing a career decision. It has also been written for senior clinicians, offering guidance and ideas about effective ways of supporting junior colleagues with their career decision-making.

Our overall aim is to provide an evidence-based approach to medical career planning. Some readers may even be surprised that there is a relevant evidence base on which to draw. Of course many areas of medical education and practice already draw heavily on psychological expertise such as the use of human factors research to enhance clinical safety and assessment theory to improve the reliability and validity of OSCEs. Yet historically, the same hasn't been true when it comes to using occupational psychology to enhance the quality of careers support provided for medical students and junior doctors. As readers of this book will find out—there is actually a wealth of relevant research that can be applied to the question of how best to plan one's medical career.

But this book—while academically robust—is also rooted in practice. One of the authors is medically qualified, and worked as a clinical director in her trust before retiring and re-training as a coach and systemic therapist. The other is an occupational psychologist and academic at a medical school, who previously set up and ran a pan-London careers support service for the London Deanery. Between them, they have provided careers support to many hundreds of medical students and qualified doctors. In addition, they have trained senior clinicians in how best to support their juniors.

We wanted to write this book because in our work we constantly encounter doctors who regret career decisions that they made in the past as well as senior clinicians who are unsure how to help students or trainees who are clearly struggling with their careers. Experience has taught us that perilously little time is devoted to career issues in the undergraduate curriculum or in later stages of training. The unspoken assumption is that medicine is a vocational degree so people have already made their career choice at the point they began the course. The fact that in the UK, there are over 60 specialties (and many more sub-specialties), is completely overlooked; the reality is that career decision-making is far from complete just because somebody has opted to study medicine, or has qualified as a doctor.

Even when somebody has chosen their specialty, their career decisions aren't finished. Specialty choice is only a small part of overall medical career planning. Some doctors may want to take their medical qualification to other countries, some have to decide if they want to follow an academic pathway, or take additional responsibilities in medical education or medical leadership. And that's just careers within the NHS. Other doctors move into private practice, or the pharmaceutical sector while a few decide that medicine in any shape or form isn't for them, and undergo more radical career shifts. Sadly a significant minority of doctors suffer burnout, and wonder what adjustments they need to make to their career, in order to make their work sustainable in the long term.

These are some of the topics that we cover in our coaching conversations with clients—conversations that we've drawn on when writing this book. So throughout the book we've combined our client experience with our analysis of relevant psychological research in order to provide a practical yet comprehensive guide to medical career planning.

Part 1 of the book provides you with a tried and tested structure broken into five stages that you can use for making career decisions at any point of your career. Perhaps five stages sounds like a lot—but as we argue in the book, your career is far too important to leave to chance. And preparing thoroughly before you make a significant career decision increases the probability that it will turn out to be a good one in the long term.

We suggest reading Part 1—or at the very least, Chapters 1 and 2—before starting on the exercises contained in these chapters. We're well aware that the prospect of career exercises might sound off-putting. But we know from our work both with individuals and groups, that people, even if initially sceptical, find these exercises hugely beneficial. The reason for this is that completing the exercises helps make people's implicit self-knowledge more explicit and in turn, this explicit knowledge can be used to make more robust career decisions. Even though we also recognize that doctors are typically time-poor, we would encourage you not to rush over the exercises—to give them the attention that they deserve.

This book has also been written for educators whose role it is to support their students or supervisees with their career planning. Educators may want to try out the exercises for themselves before recommending them to others. It's possible to engage with the exercises either as you are at your current career stage or in the role of your younger self at a time when your career path hadn't yet been established. In clinical situations, doctors are aware that simply telling patients that they need to lose weight or stop smoking is not the most effective way of getting patients to change their health beliefs or behaviour. Instead, one has to start from the understanding that the patient has of the situation, and use that as the springboard for change. In a similar way when senior doctors try to get juniors to think seriously about their career because they think the junior is making a poor career decision—giving directive advice as to what the junior doctor should do next is not the most effective method. This book will, we hope, provide senior clinicians with a practical approach to the provision of collaborative as opposed to directive career advice.

Part 2 is more varied. Chapter 9 is for the smallish number of doctors who can't seem to find any specialty that feels right—an issue that is still somewhat taboo. It's vitally important to address this issue as feeling that you are in the wrong job is distressing for the doctor, and can also impact on the quality of care given to patients. The reality is that while for many, working as a doctor is a tremendous privilege, the role doesn't suit everybody who graduates from medical school. Those considering leaving the profession need to be given an opportunity to consider the options that exist beyond clinical practice.

In contrast, everybody should read Chapter 12 which focuses on the pressures of medical work and its impact on mental health. This chapter looks critically at the realities of working as a doctor yet also provides practical and life-affirming strategies that doctors can adopt to improve their well-being.

In Chapter 13 we show that career planning is a process rather than a one-off event. The structured approach we outline has a role from the start of one's medical career right the way through to its end—and everything in between. Our advice is based upon our work as career coaches, working with those who are considering applying to medical school, those in their foundation years, doctors mid-way through training, fully qualified doctors, and those who are planning retirement.

Our hope is that by using this book, readers can side-step career regret (or can help others to do so), and instead make robust decisions leading to careers which are both rewarding and meaningful.

Additional online content

Discover downloadable templates to assist with completing the exercises and listen to podcasts containing useful tips from the authors online. Search for this book's title or ISBN (9780198884873) at https://academic.oup.com, and go to the online appendix at the end of the book.

Print readers: Use your scratch-off code on the inside cover of the book to access the material. If you would like access to the whole book, or are interested in accessing other titles, you can recommend it to your librarian.

Ebook readers: If you would like to access the book online, please recommend it to your librarian.

Online readers: Go to the online appendix at the end of the table of contents.

Steps towards a satisfying career

First steps

Imagine buying your first home. Perhaps you have done this already—or for you maybe this is something that might happen in future. Either way, what factors do you need to weigh up? Price will obviously be high up on your list, but beyond that, what else should you consider? When faced with the big purchases like a home, ideas may flow freely—location, size, character, transport links, parking, and more. Career planning is no less important than the other big decisions we make. Yet with our careers, less tangible as they seem to be, our ideas may flow less easily. Often career planning is pushed to the side or left to chance. The problem is compounded by the rigid nature of medical careers with their predefined pathways and set moments for applying for the various postgraduate training stages.

In this book we will show you a method for making career decisions in a structured way—one that's practical and won't leave you feeling anxious or confused. This chapter outlines the structure and sets about creating the cornerstone of your career planning project. The process involves nothing more complicated than thinking about yourself: your likes, needs, strengths, dislikes—as well as your areas of relative weakness. We encourage you to start the planning process as soon as possible—ideally around about the middle of your first foundation year. This gives you time both to make and to revise your career plan in the light of experiences you'll have along the way.

You already have the skills you need

It can be useful to draw a parallel between clinical decision-making and career planning. In terms of clinical decision-making, you will already be familiar with the steps, which should make it easier to apply the parallel steps when planning your career.

With clinical decision-making, history is typically the richest source of information. The same is true for career planning. Here, the most important information is the self-knowledge which emerges through guided introspection and career history review. This self-knowledge will allow you to set out what you most need from your work.

Returning to the clinical scenario, the sequence is invariably from history to physical examination. The career-planning equivalent is to progress to exploring the different specialty options that could interest you. Moving on to differential diagnosis (which if you think about it, is a kind of shortlisting process), the career-planning equivalent is to create a shortlist of potential specialty options. Continuing with the parallel, your investigations may refute some diagnoses and support others. The same is true for the investigation stage of career planning. Making self-knowledge explicit allows you to generate some targeted questions which, when answered, speak to the 'goodness of fit' between your personal needs on the one hand and the nature of the shortlisted specialties on the other. The career investigation stage involves *talking* to people in the

Table 1.1 Clinical and career planning skills

Clinical skills	Career planning skills
History	Self-knowledge
Examination	Exploration of possible options
Differential diagnosis	Shortlist of options
Investigation	Investigation
Diagnosis	Career decision
Treatment	Implementation

specialty—trainees, consultants—and if time is on your side, gaining some direct access to the specialty as well. The two final stages, diagnosis and management, translate into making your career decision and finally implementing your career plan.

The sequence shown in Table 1.1 looks rather linear. But from experience you'll know that clinical assessment is often iterative. A physical sign might lead you to recheck a historical detail. By the same token, in career planning, discovering something about a specialty can give you pause for further thought about your own interests, skills, and preferences.

All this might seem like a faff. But seriously—would you treat a patient without first carrying out some sort of assessment? Even in an emergency, you'll take a basic history and examine the patient. Your working life deserves the same level of attention.

A further benefit of being systematic shows itself at the job application stage. Having been structured, you will find yourself more articulate in the way you display your knowledge, interests, and abilities. This won't be altogether surprising given that interview panels have a need, complementary to your own, to match people to training places or jobs. So putting the time into career planning should enable both a robust career decision as well as more successful applications.

Our analogy is not perfect. The clinical scenario is usually about finding *the* correct diagnosis which will inform your treatment plan. But in the career context, the evidence suggests that each doctor could be suited to *a number* of different specialties—rather than there being only one career in which they could be happy. And another way in which our analogy is imperfect is that clinical care is intended for sick patients whereas career decision-making is for *every*body. In this sense career planning is more like a public health measure—like good nutrition or clean air. Every medical student and every doctor can benefit from a structured approach to career planning.

Preparing to carry out the exercises

We have developed the exercises in this chapter for medical students and doctors over many years. They are intended to help you build up career-relevant self-knowledge in an efficient and fine-grained way. Occasionally an exercise might lead to a tremendous insight—a eureka moment. More commonly the experience is of a gradual clarification of your ideas and of the future careers which you would enjoy. There are arguments—discussed in Box 1.1—to suggest we do better when we slow down our thinking processes. We also suggest carrying out as many of the exercises as possible. You'll benefit from a process of triangulation in which having more than one data source reduces the risk of 'error'. Each exercise works slightly differently, though they do overlap.

You may wonder if we are making a simple career decision too complicated—or if the decision is so complex that a quick, 'System 1' approach is warranted. Certainly

Box 1.1 **How we think**

Psychology and neuroscience have found compelling empirical support for the idea that much of our thinking goes on without our conscious awareness. A useful account of two contrasting thinking styles was set out by Nobel Prize winner Daniel Kahneman in his seminal book *Thinking Fast and Slow*.[1] Kahneman's 'System 1' thinking refers to our fast, automatic, and seemingly effortless way of thinking. In our slower, more effortful 'System 2' thinking, we bring rigour to some of our deliberations. We can fall prey to a variety of cognitive biases when we don't apply System 2 checks and balances to our thinking—including our career decisions.

A classic bias takes the form of the *Availability Bias* where we make a choice simply because the idea was, at the time, available in our mind. Many of us may have come into medicine because we knew more about the roles of doctors than we did about other occupational roles in healthcare or beyond. Even if this was the case and if that decision worked out well, there are still strong arguments for applying some extra checks and balances to the next leg of the journey. Kahneman suggests we impose rigorous scrutiny—or 'decision hygiene' to our decision making. In practice this means

♦ breaking decisions down into sub-decisions (stages)

♦ scoring or ranking the options under consideration

♦ delaying the use of intuition until all the information is in

There is evidence, however, that for some types of decision-making, a fast, intuitive style of thinking can be beneficial. In an ingenious series of laboratory experiments, Dijskerthuis and his team[2] asked subjects to rank the quality of different car purchases based upon their attributes: mileage, handling, age, the size of their boot, and so on. One group was also asked to perform a distracting task: one with a cognitive load that prevented them thinking about the cars in a slow, deliberate System 2 type way. Surprisingly, the distracted subjects were found to make objectively better decisions. It seems that for some complex decisions, non-conscious System 1 type processing may be important or even essential for the decision-making. For simpler decisions, i.e. rankings of hair products, or simpler car-related decisions (with fewer attributes to weigh up), slower, conscious deliberation seems to aid decision-making. David Eagleman's book *Incognito: the Secret Lives of the Brain*[3] gives a most engaging overview of some of the neuroscience.

career decisions *can* at times appear quite straightforward. But our experience has shown us that career decisions are often complex and are vulnerable to cognitive biases. Pragmatically, career theorists and career counsellors have come to the conclusion that people making career decisions should be encouraged to use both conscious and non-conscious styles of deliberation.

In this book we periodically discuss a simple rule of thumb put forward by Jonathan Haidt in his book, *The Happiness Hypothesis*.[4] Haidt uses the metaphor of a rider on top of an elephant for our conscious and non-conscious thinking: the rider, our conscious thinking, is small in comparison with the powerful elephant, our non-conscious thinking. Being smaller and weaker, the rider can guide the elephant but to a limited degree only. Should the need arise, the elephant can ignore the exhortations of the rider following her own goals and inclinations. Applying Haidt's metaphor to our work with doctors, we have sometimes observed that when a previously made career decision turned out to be at variance with a person's needs, that person came to feel they were in the wrong job. This is what happened to Tanya (Box 1.2).

Box 1.2 **Tanya and her inner elephant**

Tanya sought career coaching when she began to struggle with anxiety several years into paediatric training. Tanya always experienced a severe sinking feeling on a Sunday night and before night shifts. Tanya was well aware of her reason for choosing paediatrics. As a child, she'd lost her younger sister to leukaemia. At that point in her life she had become very accustomed to hospital environments. Tanya could see that she might have been drawn to medicine even had she and her family not suffered their devastating loss. But her experience of her sister's illness had without doubt been a factor. Despite being aware of the link, it took Tanya a great deal of introspection to see the particular effects that caring for patients had on her. In one conversation Tanya described her sense of forever being reminded of her sister's death.

To add to Tanya's confusion, the feedback she generally received was that she was very sensitive: good at working with distressed patients and their parents. In handling acute emergencies and tricky situations, Tanya was just as skilled as any doctor at compartmentalizing her own feelings. But Tanya constantly experienced a background worry about missing things and making mistakes. It became clear that this had to do with having blamed herself towards the end of her sister's short life. When her sister had been particularly ill, Tanya needed to be the model child who made few demands on her parents.

Now Tanya's elephant wanted to stampede off in a completely different direction, unwilling to continue performing the role of the model daughter/doctor. Through career coaching, it was possible to find a path for this to happen—not in an unwelcome stampede, but by identifying an interesting sub-specialty where children were less commonly as acutely unwell, so there were fewer triggers linked to her earlier experience of losing her sister.

We're not suggesting that if you have a personal or family link to a particular illness you shouldn't treat patients in the same patient group. That would be far too black and white. But what we are saying is that for *some* people, the nature of an earlier loss or illness can mean that for them it might be traumatic to treat patients with the same illness. We can free ourselves up to contemplate the issues by reviewing the stories of our lives and our careers. Sometimes we might come to realize that there may be other options we would find less traumatic, just as interesting, or better matched to our own particular set of skills, interests, and vulnerabilities.

Practicalities

Hopefully we have convinced you to talk to both your elephant and your rider. But in practice, how *can* you talk to them? Luckily, this is more straightforward than you might think. It is done simply by addressing questions about your career in a series of exercises. Though you'll always be busy, it should still be possible to carry out the exercises in moments when you are relatively relaxed. You need to be in a frame of mind to consider your strengths, weaknesses, fears, and more—as non-judgementally as possible.

Try to be organized about storing the emerging information in a private physical or virtual place. Don't try to keep the thoughts in your head where they can be forgotten or disregarded. We suggest postponing discussions with your significant others until a little later in the process. The first stage of career planning is not normally a stage to recruit help from those who may have their own ideas about the career path you should take. As for the pace, this will likely be determined by the time you have available. If time allows, it works well to complete the exercises over several months—there's no advantage in rushing.

What if I'm suffering from burnout?

The prevalence of mental illnesses such as anxiety and depression is high in both doctors and in the population at large. It goes without saying that if you are experiencing symptoms of burnout, anxiety, or depression, you deserve the best professional help available—so should seek help. In the UK, local Health Education England Professional Support Units provide career support to doctors in training. Confidential health services like Practitioner Health and DocHealth meet the mental health needs of doctors and other health professionals. We discuss such services in Chapter 12 as well as burnout and mental health more generally.

You might reasonably wonder how you can plan your career at the same time as getting help for your mental health. The short answer is that you can—but it's a question of timing. The first step is to get the right professional help and support. Then, when you feel able to do so, you can ease yourself into career planning. You'll want to factor in your feelings as well as any insights you have had along the way. For instance, you might begin to notice that a particular type of work environment, a particular pace or type of work or scenario contributes to your feelings of burnout, anxiety, or depression. If so, this knowledge could inform your subsequent career planning.

What if I have a disability?

In the UK, a person is considered to be disabled in the terms of the Equality Act 2010[5] if they have a physical or mental impairment with a substantial and long-term effect on their ability to do normal daily activities. Disability is one of the nine 'protected characteristics' under the act. But the UK regulatory body, the General Medical Council (GMC)[6] goes further, acknowledging that a disability can actually function as an asset: 'We firmly believe disabled people should be welcomed to the profession and valued for their contribution to patient care.' The GMC holds that experiencing a health condition can help a doctor to be more attuned to patients' emotional issues. Disabled doctors will have insight into their own self-care needs and the effects of their disability. Non-disabled doctors may take longer to reach a comparable level of understanding. So there are advantages which can offset any disadvantages arising from the condition itself. Another important consideration is that employers and universities have legal responsibilities to make reasonable adjustments—not only to support disabled candidates during the selection process but also, for those who are selected, to support them to reach their potential in carrying out their duties.

If you have, or think you might have a disability, you can and should feel empowered to ask for an occupational health assessment. Such an assessment should identify the areas that might be challenging for you and should suggest the kinds of adjustment you would benefit from. Consider such recommendations alongside the information that emerges from the exercises in the next chapter. Workplace adjustments and the career planning that you'll do with the aid of this book can complement each other, so that ultimately you can make a valuable contribution to a specialty that interests you and which meets your own career needs. Two very brief case studies (Box 1.3) show how this can work.

Box 1.3 Two foundation year (FY) doctors with disabilities

Rory was diagnosed with dyslexia while at university. His assessment showed that not only were spelling and reading difficult for him, but under time pressure, he also struggled with multitasking. Rory was advised about various apps that could help with spelling. He was encouraged to ask for extra time for exams and assessments that involved a fair amount of reading. But Rory realized he needed to find a specialty that wouldn't require constant multitasking under conditions of extreme time pressure. His sense was that his reading and spelling were okay compared with how much he struggled with making the transition from one activity to the next. At the exploration stage of career planning, Rory was surprised to find a number of specialty options that interested him including public health, occupational health, rehabilitation medicine, and psychiatry.

Meena has a hearing impairment and uses hearing aids supplemented by lip-reading. Her occupational health assessment recommended equipment such as an amplified stethoscope, and suggested working in quieter environments wherever possible. At the exploration stage of career planning, Meena identified various patient-facing specialties in more controllable environments, e.g. general practice, audio vestibular medicine, and clinical genetics. She also looked into specialties with little or less patient contact (such as radiology or virology) or none at all (histopathology or public health).

Summary

In this chapter, we have argued that doctors need to give career planning much greater priority. Practically, we know this is a big ask with so many demands to juggle—exams, portfolios, posts, or placements, and the need for sleep. One's own needs—especially one that seems quite distal—can so easily be set aside. But we suggest starting career planning as early as possible—so that thinking about your own needs becomes second nature. In the next chapter we introduce a series of exercises which hopefully you will enjoy and will enable you to incorporate career planning into your working life as a doctor.

References

1. **Kahneman, D.** (2011). *Thinking fast and slow*. Penguin Books.
2. **Dijksterhuis, A., Bos, M.W.,** … & **Van Baaren, R.B.** (2006). On making the right choice: the deliberation-without-attention effect. *Science*. **311**(5763):1005–1007. DOI:10.1126/science.1121629
3. **Eagleman, D.** (2016). *Incognito: the secret lives of the brain*. Canongate Books.
4. **Haidt, J.** (2006). *The happiness hypothesis*. Heinemann.
5. **Government Equalities Office and Equality and Human Rights Commission** (2015, June 16). *Equality Act 2010: guidance*. https://www.gov.uk/guidance/equality-act-2010-guidance
6. **General Medical Council** (2024). *How disability is viewed by patients, colleagues and educators*. https://www.gmc-uk.org/education/standards-guidance-and-curricula/guidance/welcomed-and-valued/how-disability-is-viewed

Further reading

Kahneman, D., Sibony, O., & Sunstein, C.R. (2022). *Noise*. William Collins.

The exercises

We will now introduce our exercises, developed through many years of working with medical students and doctors. These exercises have been designed to help clarify your own thinking. Even if you have yet to qualify, you will be surprised by the extent of your accumulated experience of being the person you are in the very many medical situations you've encountered to date. If you're already qualified with far more experience behind you, you have that much more material to review. Throughout, we encourage you to cast aside your sense of how you 'ought' to feel and to be brutally honest with yourself. In a nutshell:

Exercise 1 which takes 45 to 60 minutes, involves ranking work values from your personal perspective.

Exercise 2 which takes about an hour, involves writing down things you're proud of, both at work and in the rest of life.

Exercise 3 takes about an hour—more if you add a lot of detail. It involves making a diagram of your 'career lifeline'.

Exercise 4 takes 1 to 3 hours and is best done over more than one session. It consists of doing some autobiographical writing.

Exercise 5 which takes about 20 to 30 minutes, encourages you to draw two images! It could take considerably longer if you find you enjoy the activity.

Exercise 6 consists of logging your experiences in a simple table. It could take as little as 5 minutes for each entry, and a further 30 minutes for an overall review.

We illustrate the exercises with the reflections of some of the doctors we have coached, with their permission, and our own reflections. We discuss two further ideas integral to career planning: 'happenstance' and 'flow'. Finally, we consider how to pull your accumulated self-knowledge together in one place, ready to use for the next career-planning stage.

How to approach the exercises

We suggest carrying out as many of the exercises as possible: covering all bases. Some exercises have greater 'face validity' than others—that is to say, that you immediately understand the point and think of them as valid career tools. You may worry the experience will be repetitive. But there is value in eliciting 'redundancy'—similar information cropping up in different exercises. When we notice the same message arising from multiple sources, we should take that particular message more seriously.

The exercises can be done many times throughout your working life. Later in the book we suggest other career stages that can benefit from a return to the exercises.

Exercise 1: The values exercise

Values are beliefs that we have that are relatively enduring—though they are not necessarily immutable. It has been found that the degree of match between our own core work values and our experience of work predicts both our work performance and our job satisfaction. So it's beneficial to explore what our personal work values actually are.

One problem with the commercially available work values questionnaires is that the values don't cover some of the core aspects of medical work. To address the specific needs of doctors, Caroline, with the help of many workshop attendees, developed a medical work values tool. The values exercise works best when you can manipulate the values in real space. You can print out the page, then cut the values into 'tiles' in the way described in our case study (Box 2.1). A lower-tech method is to copy the items onto Post-It notes or slips of paper, then move them about on your tabletop.

You may wonder if you can 'eyeball the values' and reach a conclusion more quickly. To encourage you to have faith to carry out the exercise fully, we have in Box 2.1, reproduced the feedback of a doctor for whom carrying out the values exercise made a real difference.

Practically, Figure 2.1 shows the four ways in which you can categorize the values. Your task is to consider how important each value is in Figure 2.2, assigning each to an

> ### Box 2.1 **Using the values exercise**
>
> I began training in General Practice and quickly realized the specialty wasn't right for me. I felt at a loss and confused about what my options were. When it came to trying the work values exercise, I initially felt like I had travelled back to primary school: armed with scissors, I was cutting out small pieces of paper! But actually this was a real turning point for me. I found the physical act of placing the values into the various categories and seeing the result in front of me was hugely satisfying and valuable.
>
> I recall the careers questionnaire I was handed in my F2 year. In hindsight, it was limited and restrictive. This exercise felt the polar opposite. Being interactive, which worked well for me, it challenged my preconceived ideas. I was then able to talk through the results with my mentor.
>
> Deepa, ST1 in Histopathology

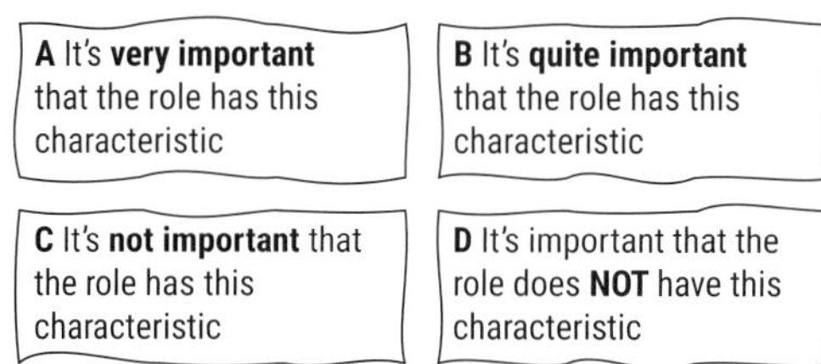

Figure 2.1 The four categories.
© Copyright Caroline Elton and Naomi Elton. Reproduced with permission.

<table>
<tr><td>

STATUS: Being highly respected by others

</td><td>

LOCATION: Being in a specific geographic place

</td></tr>
<tr><td>

EARNING WELL: Opportunity to earn a high salary

</td><td>

VARIETY of subject matter, tasks or types of patient

</td></tr>
<tr><td>

TEAMWORK: Opportunities for working as part of a team

</td><td>

FRIENDSHIP: Opportunities to develop friendships at work

</td></tr>
<tr><td>

PATIENT-FACING: Direct work with patients

</td><td>

CREATIVITY: Opportunities to create or innovate

</td></tr>
<tr><td>

AUTONOMY: Being able to determine how and when tasks are done

</td><td>

WORKING ALONE: Spending considerable time during the day on one's own

</td></tr>
<tr><td>

INTENSITY: Rapid workflow

</td><td>

COMPETITIVE: Working in a highly competitive specialty

</td></tr>
<tr><td>

Preference for certain **PATIENT TYPES**

</td><td>

Preference for certain **TECHNIQUES OR PROCEDURES**

</td></tr>
<tr><td>

EXCITING: Making high stakes decisions under pressure

</td><td>

LEADING & MANAGING people, teams, services

</td></tr>
<tr><td>

Working in a **HOSPITAL SETTING**

</td><td>

APPRECIATION: Opportunities to get positive feedback from patients and families

</td></tr>
</table>

Figure 2.2 The 36 work values. You can access a downloadable template of this figure online (search for this book's ISBN 9780198884873 at https://academic.oup.com and go to the online appendix at the end of the book. See 'Additional Online Content' for further information).

Working in a **COMMUITY SETTING**

JOB SECURITY: Plenty of training and consultant posts are likely to be available

FLEXIBLE: The culture of the speciality supports less-than-full-time working

Opportunity to provide **CONTINUITY OF CARE**

WORK-LIFE BALANCE: Not frequently working at weekends, when off duty or out-of-hours

Opportunities for **LEARNING AND DEVELOPMENT**

SUPERVISING OTHERS

HELPING individuals, community, or society

EXPERTISE: Being an acknowledged expert

PHYSICAL WORK that may be challenging

Opportunity to **BUILD COMMUNITIES**

Opportunity for **ADVANCEMENT**

PREDICTABILITY of daily/weekly routine

Opportunity for **RESEARCH** and to contribute to new developments

The specialty is likely to offer **NEW CHALLENGES** in the future

Working in a nationally or internationally recognised **INSTITUTE**

Opportunities to **TEACH** and train others

Predominantly **DETAILED** work

Figure 2.2 Continued

importance category. You can change your mind as much as you want. Try not to place *all* the values into one category, unless you're sure this is how you really feel.

Ranking the values

The next stage is to rank-order the values you have already categorized.

1. Re-consider the values in Category A (Very important) and Category B (Quite important). With their importance in mind, rank-order them into *one* list of descending importance. The values in Categories A and B may now mix up. We suggest your top eight values are particularly important—but you may prefer to retain more or less than this number for later consideration.

2. Re-consider the values in Category D (Important not-to-have). Rank-order these into one list of descending importance *not* to have that value. We suggest retaining a smaller number of values—around three—but again, the number is your choice.

3. Re-consider the values in Category C (Not important). If they still seem unimportant, discard them.

4. Note your rank-ordered lists using Table 2.1 and Table 2.2 (or something similar).

You may wonder how necessary it is to commit your rankings to writing. It's tempting to rely on memory but writing down your rankings takes only a minute. Doing so doesn't commit you to them but helps you recall the detail which may evade you once you embark on the subsequent exercises.

More exercises are necessary because it would be a lot to expect that one exercise alone could tell you which specialty to choose. Knowing your own values is just *the*

Table 2.1 'Very important' and 'Quite important' values. You can access a downloadable template of this table online (search for this book's ISBN 9780198884873 at https://academic.oup.com and go to the online appendix at the end of the book. See 'Additional Online Content' for further information). © Copyright Caroline Elton and Naomi Elton. Reproduced with permission.

Most important values	
1st most important	
2nd most important	
3rd most important	
4th most important	
5th most important	
6th most important	
7th most important	
8th most important	

Table 2.2 'Important-not-to-have' values. You can access a downloadable template of this table online (search for this book's ISBN 9780198884873 at https://acade mic.oup.com and go to the online appendix at the end of the book. See 'Additional Online Content' for further information). © Copyright Caroline Elton and Naomi Elton. Reproduced with permission.

Most important-*not-to-have* values	
1st most important-*not-to-have*	
2nd most important-*not-to-have*	
3rd most important-*not-to-have*	

start of the journey. It is important to resist the temptation to look into specialty destinations right away. The clearer you are about your career needs *before* exploring the specialties, the more effective will be the process of exploration.

Some further reflections

◆ Did anything surprise you? Or did the exercise confirm preferences you already knew you had? Even in the latter case it's helpful to notice any prior knowledge, now validated through the exercise.

◆ It's possible (though not necessarily easy) to conjure up your hopes for the future—perhaps travelling, or having a family. At the point of starting a family, location can become that much more important. It is more common for women than men to work less-than-full-time after childbearing but there is considerable variation in how many hours are worked.[1] Can you sense how you might rank values like these in future?

◆ Has a value cropped up, the importance of which is very great, but which you think cannot be fulfilled through working as a doctor? Should you find yourself recognizing this scenario, do you think it may be sufficient for you to find an outlet for that important value outside work? If after much careful thought the answer to this is also negative, the remaining self-knowledge exercises will be especially important to you. Some, but by no means all doctors in this position will also find Chapter 9 helpful.

Exercise 2: Achievements

It's often said that we should play to our strengths. But medical culture can make this hard. Understandably, portfolios encourage reflection of episodes that went less well. And the fast pace of medical life can be such that there's little time to dwell on the successes. New challenges come thick and fast, requiring your full attention.

It's possible though, to deepen your understanding of yourself and what motivates you by thinking about things that went well. This exercise invites you to dwell

Box 2.2 **An achievement of Caroline's**

A moment of pride that springs to mind is working with a particular doctor, Estelle, to identify a satisfying career beyond medicine. Estelle had been diagnosed with schizophrenia when still at medical school. Her condition was relatively well managed with medication, and she was successful in gaining her medical degree, though it took her a number of extra years to do so. Estelle went on to find the responsibility of working as a foundation doctor overwhelming. It was clear to her supervisors that continuing up the career ladder would be unlikely to work out for Estelle.

Helping Estelle to come to terms with the sense of medicine not now being right for her—and identifying a more suitable career pathway was incredibly challenging. But seeing her able to move on, and over time, to make a success of her new non-medical career meant a huge amount to me. This example made me realize that client work is at the heart of what I do—and I would not be happy in a job that didn't allow me to work with clients, at least some of the time.

immodestly on your successes. We suggest you identify two or three achievements in work or training that make you feel particularly proud, and a similar number of examples from outside work. When choosing, don't select the grand achievements you would include in an application. More important may be the smaller details within the achievements that gave you a particular sense of fulfilment. They might seem quite ordinary to other people. The important thing is that they really mattered to you.

In Box 2.2, Caroline talks about an achievement in her own career. We use Box 2.3 to outline a case study in which Harri, an F1 doctor used an achievement for career planning. Inevitably, our case studies oversimplify things. In reality Harri would have carried out many more of the exercises.

For each of your achievements, consider

◆ Why you chose this particular achievement from the many possibilities. What does this particular choice say about what's important to you?

◆ To achieve these things, which of your skills and abilities did you draw upon?

◆ For this achievement, how did you relate to others? To what extent did you work closely with others, lead others, follow others, or work on your own?

◆ How does this particular achievement fit with what you know about your personality, your upbringing, your role models, and your life experience?

◆ What feedback did you receive from others about the achievement?

◆ Consider a person who knows you well and whose opinion you value. What might they say about this achievement? What would they consider it to say about you?

◆ Taking into account all of these points, what are your areas of real strength that you would like to build upon in your future job role?

> ### Box 2.3 F1 doctor's experience with the achievements exercise
>
> Harri, an F1 doctor, remembered a role several years earlier when he worked as a volunteer at a summer camp for disabled children. He recalled how happy he'd been to find he could relate well to the children and young people. A crisis had occurred when a group of teenagers went missing. Harri's team leader had praised his personal skills in that situation. At the time, Harri had felt he had done well to escalate the situation while personally remaining involved. He'd supported the senior staff who had seemed super-stressed. Reflecting on the incident as part of the exercise, Harri realized how well he could solve problems, even under duress.
>
> In relation to work, Harri, considered his contribution in the Covid19 pandemic as a personal achievement. The ward had, at times, been truly chaotic. Harri reflected that he had made sure to look out for colleagues, checking if they were okay. Harri found himself speaking for his cohort of foundation doctors. Others had appreciated it when he had voiced the group's concerns.
>
> Harri realized that the skills he wanted to build on in his future career included problem-solving, working under pressure, teamwork, and his ability to notice and respond to what was happening around him. He looked forward to one day leading a team. He also realized how much he enjoyed working with children.

Take-away messages

Once again, note down in a few bullet points, the high-level messages that you want to take from the achievements exercise. This might be about what motivates you or in what sort of environment you work best. Or it might be about what others have fed back to you about your achievements.

Exercise 3: Career lifeline

The career lifeline exercise tends to appeal to those whose thinking is aided by something visual. The aim is to construct a diagram of your career so far. Turn an A4 page to landscape and draw a horizontal from one side to the other about halfway down the page. Next, chart your career visually as an ascending and descending line from your senior school years at one side, progressing to the present at the other. Place experiences with an overall positive feel above the line and those with an overall negative feel below. It can be hard to choose, particularly if (as is often the case) the experience was mixed. Rating an experience negatively can feel disloyal but consider that this a private and highly subjective aid to thinking.

Next, add some commentary: some detail about what the experiences felt like. You may need to make several revisions as Naomi did for her career lifeline shown in Figure 2.3, discussed in Box 2.4.

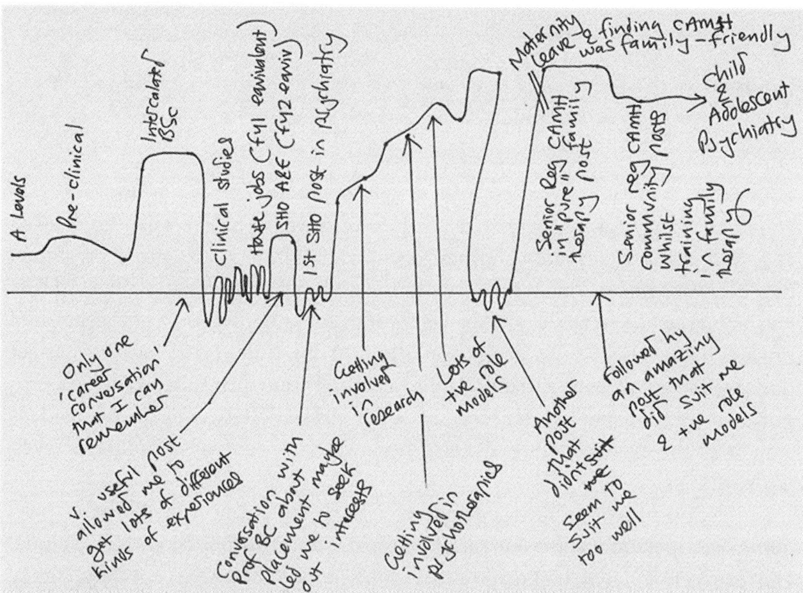

Figure 2.3 Naomi's career lifeline.

Box 2.4 Reflections arising from Naomi's career lifeline

Making a career lifeline showed me how important it had been to follow my interests. I felt more engaged during my psychology BSc year than when studying other preclinical subjects. For those more 'negative' studies, I seemed to be motivated by fear of failure. After my intercalated BSc, I considered switching to psychology but continued with medicine. After house jobs (equivalent to F1), I did a stint as senior house officer (SHO) in A&E. I wanted to double check if psychiatry was right for me. In A&E, I revelled in activities like suturing in 'minors' but dreaded some of the more complicated 'majors'—except for 'overdoses' for which I was the go-to SHO. Confirming this area of interest helped validate my choice to train in psychiatry.

I seemed to take it quite hard when a particular post didn't suit me. Typically, in-patient psychiatric settings were not my bag. I preferred the autonomy of out-patient work and was particularly drawn to the psychotherapies. I had some wonderful role models—psychiatrists who were also talented family therapists. Looking back though, I can see how few career conversations I had with my role models! These sorts of conversations were generally had with peers. I think I placed the seniors on a pedestal far too much. I was wary of sharing my hopes and dreams with them, perhaps for good reason as there was a quite an authoritarian culture at the time. My inner 'elephant' however, found ingenious solutions—to train in systemic therapy and later in occupational psychology.

CAMHS became the family-friendly specialty of choice for me. As a child psychiatrist, I was fascinated by the gentle (and sometimes not-so-gentle) dramas that unfolded when working with families. I felt most fulfilled when I could put parents to good use in supporting their teenager's recovery.

The prompts here are to aid reflection:

◆ What do the positively and negatively rated experiences say about you and about your preferences?

◆ What kinds of experiences did you find sufficiently fulfilling to want more of them? What were the most important elements without which the overall experience would have been less good?

◆ What experiences were particularly stressful to you? What elements made them stressful? How likely is it that you would deal with similar stressors in the same way if they were to recur? Are there any stressors that are important to avoid for the future?

Each career lifeline is unique. The lifeline exercise may help you spot something you had previously overlooked. If the exercise tells you something you already knew, try to welcome the repetition as valuable intelligence. You can also use your lifeline to consider *how* you made the choices that you made. You might notice that you made some of your decisions analytically. Other decisions may have been made by virtue of having been 'in the right place at the right time'. Or because you had a particular conversation with a particular person.

The haphazard nature of career decisions was noticed by career theorist, John Krumboltz who provided a useful counterbalance to the then popular psychometric testing that dominated career guidance. Krumboltz contended that careers don't always follow logical or planned paths.[2] Alongside the structured approach to career planning that we outline in this book, Krumboltz argued that we need to take advantage of unexpected opportunities that arise. We might think of opportunities as applying more to entrepreneurs than doctors, but opportunities can arise for any of us at any career stage. Caroline is neither an entrepreneur nor a doctor but her career-shape illustrates this point (Box 2.5).

Take-away messages

Take a moment to note the main messages arising from the lifeline exercise. Comment on the sorts of condition you thrive in, what seems to cause you stress, what opportunities presented themselves to you and how you responded.

Exercise 4: The writing exercise

Recall Haidt's 'Elephant and the rider' and the need to factor both into the making of complex decisions. Writing can be a surprisingly effective way to access the elephant's experience. The act of writing seems to release the flow of ideas, somewhat altering our habitual ways of thinking. In conversation, we can easily censor our ideas. Pondering on our own, we might go round in circles. A similar liberation from such habits can occur with drawing and other forms of creative expression.

Use a blank page to write about your career—an account that is for your eyes only. The writing can be free-style—or could take the form of an unsent letter to a significant person, alive or dead, or to your past or your future self. If you feel able, write about your career without using the following prompts. If you prefer,

> ## Box 2.5 Planned happenstance in Caroline's career
>
> A year or so into my part-time PhD, I hit a roadblock. Recruiting patients into the sample was slower than I'd originally anticipated. I now needed to widen my net by recruiting patients from a larger number of hospitals. Applying to the research ethics committees of the additional hospitals took time, and having already written my literature review, I was stuck.
>
> One day I happened upon an advert for a part-time job as an education adviser working locally. In some ways it was a step backwards as I had left teaching to train in psychology. But it looked interesting, so I decided to apply and was duly appointed. It was supposed to be for six months but in the end the contract was extended and I did it for three years, alongside my part-time PhD.
>
> When I finished my PhD I wasn't sure what to do next. I hadn't planned to work in medical education, but I happened to see another job advert for a medical education adviser working with one of the postgraduate deaneries. You needed a PhD (which I'd just finished), and you needed to be a teacher (which I had been in the past). And the icing on the cake was that you also needed experience of educational advisory work. By chance—because of the part-time job I did when my PhD had hit the roadblock, I could tick that box as well. I applied, and over 20 years later, while I'm not still in the same role, I still work in medical education.
>
> Looking back, the key was being willing to give something different a try. When an unexpected opportunity arose, I could have thought, 'It's a step backwards and not what I'm planning to do, so I'll ignore it' but instead, I asked myself if it might work out. The 'happenstance' bit was that these two different random opportunities arose. The 'planned' bit was that I had a pretty good understanding of what I enjoyed doing, what I was good at, what I was hopeless at, and what was most important to me in my work.

go through the prompts one at a time but try to write in whole sentences like this one rather than bullet points (as follows) in your own writing. Doing so may help you reflect.

- What were the most influential episodes at work or outside work?
- If you haven't already done so, write about your achievements and the small moments that gave you great satisfaction or meant a lot to you.
- Write about those who influenced you (your role models) in both positive and negative ways.
- Reflect on your upbringing, the careers of family members, which career was expected for you (or which you expected) and how you responded to any expectations.
- How did you discover your core values?

- What ambitions have you had over time? Who or what helped you achieve your ambitions? What barriers have you experienced?
- Why do you think things happened the way they did?
- What do you enjoy the most? What causes you stress?
- Keeping in mind that everybody makes mistakes, what mistakes did you make?
- How would you describe the career dilemmas you now face?
- What opportunities may lie ahead?

Take-away messages

Writing can be absorbing or it can feel like a chore. Either way, it's helpful to put the piece to one side, approaching it afresh a day or two later. You may then feel compelled to add to what you've already written. You can also highlight what seems important. If you notice repetition, it's worth wondering why it might have been important to re-state that point. Do you notice any changes in what seemed important to you as time went on? Does anything surprise you? What seems particularly typical of yourself?

Overall, what few points do you feel are the most important to take away? Try to be disciplined and note them.

Exercise 5: The drawing exercise

Many of us feel wary of drawing (although some doctors, like our illustrator Paula, are excellent artists). Before dismissing the idea of drawing, consider that an image could tap into deeper ideas with less filtering. When you feel courageous, take a large sheet of paper and give yourself free rein to create an image conveying something about your *current* work. This could take 20 minutes or longer. There are no rules about how it should look. As the drawing is for you alone, it doesn't have to be artistic: it can be diagrammatic, abstract, simple, or comprehensive. It can feature stick figures, be coloured-in, or consist only of outlines.

We suggest making a second image representing how you want your work to be *in the future*. Jade, our case study, discussed in Box 2.6, gave us permission to reproduce her drawing shown in Figure 2.4.

Take-away messages

As with the writing exercise, we recommend returning to your creation with fresh eyes in a day or two.

- What do you observe?
- What do you make of the colours or style?
- What about the content? What seems important?
- What do you think your younger self might make of what you've put down on paper? What about your older, wiser self?

Note the key points you would like to take from the exercise.

> ## Box 2.6 Drawing can give you courage
>
> Jade, an ST5 in O&G, was working flat-out throughout her first pregnancy and feeling pretty exhausted. Jade drew herself, roller-skating from room to room, dripping with sweat.
>
> The image that represented Jade's work 5 years into the future showed Jade, her partner, and child standing near their house, also near Jade's hospital and the sea. In the picture Jade was teaching yoga to some pregnant women. Creating this image helped Jade to 'own' an idea she had been turning over in her mind—something she wanted to do.
>
> Jade undertook training in yoga instruction, developed her networks, and found a business partner. After maternity leave, she took time out of training to develop the ideas further, before returning to train and gaining her Certificate of Completion of Training (CCT).

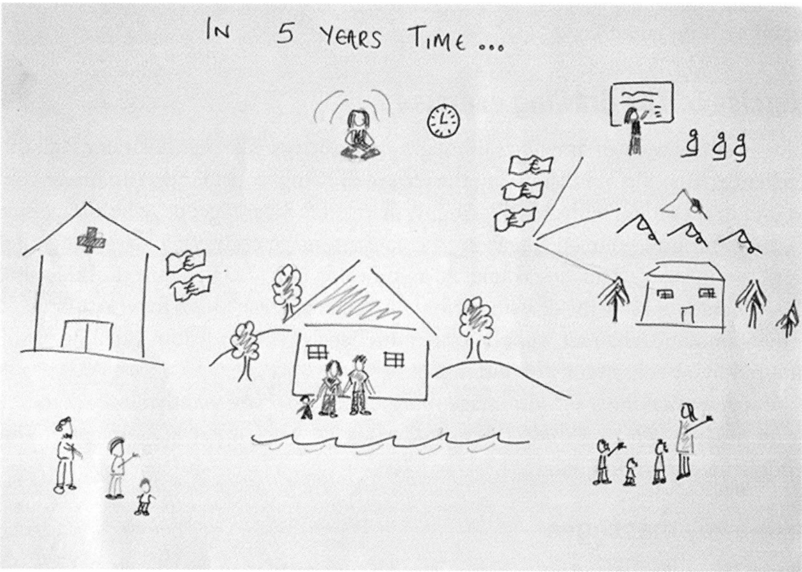

Figure 2.4 Jade's possible future.

Exercise 6: Experience log

Some of the foregoing exercises (the writing, your career lifeline and your achievements) relied on recalling past events. A prospective log, made soon after episodes occur, can complement that approach. A log might feel similar to your training e-portfolio, but this is a private log with a different purpose. It aims to help clarify your thoughts and feelings about the elements that make up your work (or your experiences

Table 2.3 Jo's experience log. You can access a downloadable template of this table online (search for this book's ISBN 9780198884873 at https://academic.oup.com and go to the online appendix at the end of the book. See 'Additional Online Content' for further information).

Experience log			
When?	**Activity you carried out as part of your job role. Include as much detail as you want**	**How would you describe your feelings during or after this activity?**	**0–10 rating (above 5 = positive below 5 = negative emotions)**	**What may be important about this for your future?**
29 May	Reading a couple of articles (updates about clinical stuff) after blood results & processing incoming letters	Desperate, asking myself why am I doing this?	-10 (off the scale)	I REALLY need to do the continuous professional development (CPD) but at a different time
1 June	Seeing a baby with chronic nappy rash	Surprisingly enjoyable	9	Being a parent has changed my perspective, I now know how much parents worry and feel so much more competent with parents and children
8 June	Treating a young man with antibiotics for a chest infection	Accomplishment	8	I didn't realize before how important it is for me to get people better relatively quickly. Perhaps this really is something that's more possible in GP than other specialties
9 June	A case discussion in the staff room, there were complex safeguarding concerns	Anxious, relieved this wasn't my patient	3	Would feel more confident if I'd seen more cases like this before. Doesn't put me off GP (all specialties have safeguarding. I'd be inhuman if I wasn't anxious)

outside work). Here, experiences that frustrate you, that seem pointless, or that you dislike are just as important to recognize as those that demonstrate your strengths and abilities.

Use a blank version of Table 2.3. Try to restrict yourself to a short comment for each entry as the aim is to collect around 20 episodes over a few weeks to allow

> ### Box 2.7 **Jo's heartening experience log**
>
> Several years after her CCT (Certificate of Completion of Training) in General Practice, Jo was feeling particularly stressed. In the week, her husband was in a city 70 miles away, finishing his clinical fellowship. Jo doubled up as a solo parent and less-than-full-time (LTFT) GP. Jo knew things would improve once her husband was working closer to home but first he had to be appointed to a consultant post. It would be amazing if this could be somewhere near to his parents who could then help with the childcare.
>
> Jo was massively sleep-deprived. She knew pulling out her work laptop when the children were asleep wasn't great for her well-being. But she really needed to check the blood results, make referrals, and do some reading to update herself about various clinical topics. The breadth of the subject matter to keep up with made Jo wonder if general practice was really right for her.
>
> The prospect of logging experiences wasn't appealing but Jo found it took just a few minutes. Surprisingly, Jo found there was a lot of positivity which seemed to be associated with a wide variety of clinical situations. The negatives had to do with the juggling that occurred in the week—trying to get things done (especially the reading) when tired. Experience logging triggered some new time management ideas as well as some options to consider within general practice.

patterns to emerge. You can carry out the exercise multiple times in different placements. Once you start, you may be surprised by the variety of experiences you log. We illustrate this point with a case study, Jo, a General Practice trainee (Box 2.7 and Table 2.3).

Bear in mind that that the learning of new skills inevitably brings a degree of emotional pain. So if you find yourself recording negative reactions—as in the case study (Box 2.7), consider that you might feel differently as you gain more experience and become more skilled.

In Box 2.8, Naomi discusses her own use of the experience log at a decision-point in her own career.

Take-away messages

You can see that the experience log is good for finding out what's going on for you, whatever your career stage.

- In your own experience log, does any kind of pattern emerge?
- Does any entry alert you to something important about your experience of work?
- What does the log tell you about what kind of person you are when at work?
- What does it tell you about your needs and preferences?
- What does it tell you about the kind of team and people you like working with?
- Is there a type of activity you could not do without?

- Do you notice any *flow activities* (discussed in Box 2.9)? If so, what might this suggest for your future career?
- Do any of your entries speak to your strengths and weaknesses? If so, how might these inform your future career choices?
- Did you log any activities that you would happily jettison if you could?
- Consider emotions like fear, anxiety, and worry associated with particular tasks. These can lessen with greater experience and practice of the relevant skills. Has this generally been the case for you?

Looking at your experience log in its entirety, try to note the most important takeaway points.

Box 2.8 **Naomi's use of the experience log**

I reached the dizzy height of clinical director in my NHS trust. Finally I could prove something to myself and others! Through grafting I have usually been able to achieve what I've wanted, though at a cost. This role was no exception but I also knew the role was 'not really me'. I found myself wide awake at night, problem-solving to the point of keeping a notebook by the bedside—just in case of a eureka moment.

Alongside the management work, I kept far more clinical work ticking over than was wise. Why did I resist giving up the clinics? I rationalized it was impossible to find the locum cover I would need to be able to do fewer clinics myself. But when I logged my experiences I discovered (what, in truth I already knew)—that what I found most fulfilling was having meaningful contact with patients, their families, or with an individual like a mentee. I did get a buzz from constructing new business plans and problem-solving the thorny issues we seemed to have. But I didn't enjoy the many routine meetings in which key performance indicators were discussed at length in meetings that chuntered through interminable agendas. These meetings were generally held in charmless meeting rooms. I wasn't always adequately prepared. The stress associated with the speed-reading (particularly when it came to interrogating excel spreadsheets) jumped out at me in my own experience log.

When the opportunity arose to re-apply for my management role, I chose instead to return to clinical practice.

What about personality questionnaires?

It's logical to wonder if personality testing can help with career planning. Personality questionnaires reveal how extraverted or introverted we are, our tendency to worry, how conscientious we are, and so on. Some studies of doctors find some personality types to be more prevalent in some specialties.[5] But it's also the case that most personality types are seen in most specialties.[6] Moreover, job satisfaction does not appear to be greater if your personality is more similar to those people commonly encountered

> ## Box 2.9 **Flow activities**
>
> The concept of flow was developed by psychologist Mihaly Csikszentmihalyi who interviewed numerous creative individuals—composers, dancers as well as chess players—asking them about their bursts of productivity.[3,4] A description that kept cropping up was that of being totally absorbed in an activity that was intrinsically enjoyable. This is what he termed 'flow'.
>
> The experience of flow is of being alert and focussed. When flow occurs, the passage of time (the past, the future) and one's own 'ego-related thoughts' cease to be important. Flow is associated with a feeling of great satisfaction.
>
> There are several important necessary conditions for flow:
>
> - Feeling in control
> - The activity is done 'for its own sake', not solely for external reasons
> - The activity is difficult but is not so difficult that it exceeds the person's skill
> - The activity has clear, intrinsic short-term goals
> - Within the activity, immediate feedback allows the person to know how they are doing
>
> Flow can be experienced in many contexts. Sadly, for some people, the only recreational flow activity they can describe is driving a motor vehicle. At work, typical examples include talking through and solving problems, completing paperwork to one's satisfaction or mending equipment. *Many* of the tasks carried out by doctors (and other clinicians) have the potential to be experienced as flow activities.

in a particular specialty.[7] But your personality may influence *how* you approach your job role; an extraverted doctor might particularly enjoy giving presentations or teaching large groups while somebody more introverted might gain more satisfaction from giving 1:1 supervision. But it's not clearcut. Many of us learn a range of strategies to allow us to rise to many challenges. Extraverts and introverts (and those in the middle) are needed across all specialties.

Personality is important, but there isn't a clear way to match medical specialties and personalities. Our approach is not to measure personality but to allow your personality to freely influence the way you respond in the exercises and thus to guide your career decisions.

Pulling the information together

You'll by now have collected a substantial body of information about yourself: the take-away messages from each exercise. The next step is to set out all these messages in one place. In addition, if you have benefited from any other assessments—such as an occupational health assessment, it's helpful also to include any recommendations you have been given.

Table 2.4 Pulling the information together. You can access a downloadable template of this table online (search for this book's ISBN 9780198884873 at https://acade mic.oup.com and go to the online appendix at the end of the book. See 'Additional Online Content' for further information). © Copyright Caroline Elton and Naomi Elton. Reproduced with permission.

Essential criteria The specialty role *must* allow for . . .	Desirable criteria It would be nice if the specialty role allowed for . . .

Table 2.5 A simpler format. You can access a downloadable template of this table online (search for this book's ISBN 9780198884873 at https://academic.oup.com and go to the online appendix at the end of the book. See 'Additional Online Content' for further information). © Copyright Caroline Elton and Naomi Elton. Reproduced with permission.

Criteria The specialty role should allow for:

We suggest using Table 2.4 or one similar to organize the elements you consider important for your future career into essential and desirable criteria for work. You will recognize that this is the same format as that commonly used in person specifications. There is one obvious difference: instead of the criteria being used to judge applicants, here they will be used to assist *you* in judging job roles or specialty options. In the next chapter we discuss our rationale for borrowing from the world of recruitment. If you find it hard to make a distinction between essential and desirable criteria, you can create just one set of criteria shown in Table 2.5.

A case study—that of Sam, an F3 doctor, discussed in Box 2.10 and Table 2.6 illustrates the approach. To cut to the chase, in his shortlisting process (to be discussed in Chapter 3), Sam selected Ear, Nose, and Throat (ENT), Ophthalmology, Orthopaedics, and Radiology.

Box 2.10 **Sam's use of the exercises**

Sam, an 'F3' doctor reviewed his career from his GCSEs onwards. At school he had loved art including textiles. The achievements exercise saw him describe himself as practical, intelligent, and creative. As a school student he had raised funds for a charity. At medical school Sam had been talented at searching out cutting edge research and intriguing resources for problem-based learning. In the values exercise, Sam identified the importance to him of being hospital-based, working in a multidisciplinary team and working with just one bodily system or clinical area.

Sam decided to complete the experience log considering each of the posts he had already done retrospectively. Doing so helped him realize the immense satisfaction he gained from performing practical procedures, especially if the procedure made an immediate difference to a patient. Something as simple as removing a foreign body from the eye had made him feel 'disproportionately fulfilled'. At the time he had dismissed his feeling of pride, noticing that nobody seemed particularly impressed. But Sam now considered that even the steps of putting the patient at their ease, explaining what would happen had all given him satisfaction. In contrast, he had felt frustrated with the 'long, tedious ward rounds' in psychiatry.

Table 2.6 Information pulled together

Essential Criteria What the specialty role *must* allow (or must not allow)	Desirable criteria It would be nice if the specialty role allowed (or did not allow)
Hospital based	Possibility of run-through training
Multidisciplinary training (MDT) working	Option to specialize in shorter procedures/operations
Procedures	Option for later private practice
Ability to specialize on one system or part of the body	Option for flexible working
Must see the effects of interventions on patients' quality of life	

Contrast Sam with Chris, immersed in his F2 psychiatric placement, discussed in Box 2.11 and Table 2.7 and who we will discuss further in the next chapter.

Summary

You will by now be familiar with the idea that different exercises throw up different (though complementary) aspects of your work in medicine. Seeing similar

Box 2.11 **F2 doctor's use of the exercises**

Chris had constructed his career lifeline, annotating it in detail. Previously Chris had been into music but had given up playing at university. He'd enjoyed his time at medical school but felt frustrated that some topics hadn't been covered in sufficient depth—topics like psychosomatic medicine, general practice, and epidemiology.

Chris carried out his experience log prospectively during the psychiatry part of his F2 year. He noted moments when talking to patients about their lives seemed to be the most meaningful experience he had had in recent years. But Chris found the structure of the psychiatric interview frustrating. He was keen to experiment with more creative ways of working with patients. Nonetheless, Chris was astonished that in the ward rounds, so much expertise was brought together from the work of each team-member. The non-psychiatric aspects of the work—like being asked to interpret electrocardiogram (ECGs) engendered mixed feelings. Chris felt perplexed that consultants left the interpretation of ECGs to F2 doctors. This led Chris to wonder if going down the psychiatric route might 'waste the medical knowledge' he had accumulated. We'll return to Chris in Chapter 3 but first, we'll look at his criteria.

Table 2.7 Information pulled together

Criteria
History taking is what I enjoy most—being able to work in not too hurried a way
Want to be able to understand patients' illnesses in the context of their lives
Work meaningfully with relatives as well as patients
Get out of hospitals, at least for part of the time
Prefer working with adult patients
Job role's security is important
Feel stimulated by MDT working—v rewarding and social

information coming from different angles can help you give serious consideration to that information.

As you proceed, you will find that some aspects of your work in medicine are sufficiently important to include them in your list of personal criteria. These criteria can now assist you in weighing up whether a specialty could meet your needs. It's tempting not to write anything down. But you are not writing it in stone. You can always change your criteria as you gain additional experience. Sometimes uncovering more information about the specialties in the next stage—the exploration stage—may turn some of your ideas on their head. You may then deprioritize something you had previously considered important—or the opposite can occur. Either way, a clear understanding of oneself is the cornerstone of robust career planning.

Additional downloadable content

Downloadable templates to assist you when undertaking the exercises and podcasts voiced by the authors are available online. Search for this book's ISBN (9780198884873) at https://academic.oup.com and go to the online appendix at the end of the book. See 'Additional Online Content' for further information.

References

1. **Kelly, E & Stockton, I.** (2022). *Working patterns of doctors and nurses returning from maternity leave.* Institute for Fiscal Studies. https://ifs.org.uk/articles/working-patterns-doctors-and-nurses-returning-maternity-leave

2. **Krumboltz, J.D.** (2009). The happenstance learning theory. *J Career Assess.* **17**(2):135–154. https://doi.org/10.1177/1069072708328861

3. **Csikszentmihalyi, M., & LeFevre, J.** (1989). Optimal experience in work and leisure. *J Pers Soc Psychol.* **56**(5). https://doi.org/10.1037/0022-3514.56.5.815

4. **Csikszentmihalyi, M.** (1999). If we are so rich, why aren't we happy?. *Am Psychol.* **54**(10):821–827. https://doi.org/10.1037/0003-066X.54.10.821

5. **Mullola, S., Hakulinen, C., … & Elovainio, M.** (2018). Personality traits and career choices among physicians in Finland: employment sector, clinical patient contact, specialty and change of specialty. *BMC Med Educ.* **18**:1–12. https://doi.org/10.1186/s12909-018-1155-9

6. **Borges, N.J., & Savickas, M.L.** (2002). Personality and medical specialty choice: a literature review and integration. *J Career Assess.* **10**(3):362–380. https://doi.org/10.1177/106727 02010003006

7. **Sievert, M., Zwir, I., … & Cloninger, C.R.** (2016). The influence of temperament and character profiles on specialty choice and well-being in medical residents. *PeerJ.* **4**:e2319. DOI: 10.7717/peerj.2319

Chapter 3

Exploring the options

We've now arrived at the exploration phase of career planning. You may feel that the self-knowledge stage entailed plenty of exploration but here you turn from looking inwardly at yourself to the 'out there' world of career options. A temptation may arise to veer off in different directions—which can quickly lead to feeling overwhelmed. To guard against this, we re-visit the concept of decision hygiene and illustrate our approach by first reviewing how organizations select *people* for *posts*. In fact, borrowing some of the language and methods from selection panels can be useful in the context of exploring career options. We then go on to discuss where to find the information you need about the various specialty options as well as how to process the information you gather, in order to make sense of it all.

Why be systematic?

There are many reasons why we encourage you to explore as widely and as systematically as you can. Firstly, of course, your specialty choice is one of the bigger life decisions you'll make—one you may live with for your whole working life. Secondly, if you consider that there are over 60 specialties, you're unlikely to have been exposed to all that could be worth considering. The undergraduate curriculum is so full that many specialties inevitably remain invisible to medical students. These tend to be the more specialized areas of medicine in which it would be hard to find meaningful medical student roles, so these specialities are typically encountered after qualifying. But with practical limits to the number of placements in foundation posts, you may not have encountered them in your foundation years either. And when it comes to international medical graduates, in many countries the intern or resident period is just one year long making exposure to some of the smaller specialties even less likely for this group of doctors.

In Chapter 2 we encouraged you to use 'decision hygiene' in the sense of using the exercises to collect information about yourself, your needs, strengths, and stress-points. Now, as we shift the spotlight to the world of opportunities, we adhere to a similar approach. Decision hygiene encourages us to break bigger decisions into smaller steps, to score and rank options—and to deploy your intuitive thinking only when sufficient information has been gathered.

Seeing the world through recruiters' eyes

To introduce our method, we will first stray into the world of recruiters.

The process of selecting people for job roles has been the subject of considerable psychological research. Thirty years ago, if you wanted to apply for a training post,

Table 3.1 Score sheet for applicants A, B, and C

	Applicant A	Applicant B	Applicant C
Application form score			
Exam score			
Interview score			
Total score			

you sent off a CV or completed an application form. If you were shortlisted, you were interviewed. Nowadays these earlier approaches to selection have now mostly been superseded by structured and standardized methods such as multiple mini interviews, designed to be objective and therefore fairer.

There's an important reason for these shifts in approach. When employees' future performance on the job has been used as the criterion for judging, structured interviews have been found to predict future performance more accurately than the traditional unstructured interview.[1,2] In contrast, when unstructured assessment interviews without rating guidelines have been used, the assessors' thinking tended to be influenced by cognitive shortcuts including the stereotyping of applicants. In other words, unconscious biases are given free rein. You may wonder, what this could have to do with you and your own exploration. Our reasoning is that just as decision hygiene is helpful in selecting people for jobs, it can also be helpful to select *jobs* for *people*.

The parallel becomes clearer if we perform a simple thought-experiment. Table 3.1 illustrates Applicants A, B, and C, to be judged for one job using three selection methods: the application form, an exam, and an interview. By completing a score sheet, the panel members can compare the applicants at a glance.

Our suggestion is that you do the same for the specialties you identify in your exploration as being worthy of consideration. You'll see from Table 3.2 that our suggested score sheet follows the same format as the applicant score sheets used by selection panels. Instead of comparing applicants, the comparison is between the specialty options. The rows for the different selection methods are replaced by your personal criteria for work—those discussed in Chapter 2. The number or rows and columns will vary. And of course, it's not essential to use a table of numerical scores. You may prefer to use narrative comments in a format that allows comparison. What's important is to be systematic.

Sources of information about specialties

Many sources of information are available to you. We caution against relying on your prior knowledge of specialties. Instead we would encourage you to *research* each option more systematically.

Table 3.2 Score sheet for specialties A, B, and C

	Specialty A	Specialty B	Specialty C
Criterion 1 Specialty must allow me to . . .			
Criterion 2 Specialty is concerned with . . .			
Criterion 3 Specialty does not involve . . .			
Criterion 4 The consultant is likely to . . .			
Total score			

The official websites

In the UK, all the specialties are listed on a website hosted by Health Education England (HEE). The list includes the training routes, eligibility criteria, selection criteria. Competition Ratios (discussed further in Chapter 6) are also published—the number of applicants per post in recent years. We have listed the main websites at the end of the chapter—with the caveat that websites and the official bodies hosting them do change.

When searching for information online, select information from the most credible source. The royal colleges, responsible for postgraduate education and training standards, provide detailed descriptions about the specialties and training routes. Each royal college formats the information differently.

Unofficial sources of information

Another approach is to seek the opinions of authors through their blogs, vlogs, papers, and books like, for example, *So You Want To Be a Brain Surgeon.*[3] Books can save a lot of time as the authors try to set out the information about the different specialties consistently. As we ourselves can attest to, book authors enjoy greater independence than do the authors of the official websites. While books and websites can become out-of-date, the 'official' websites are likely to be updated more frequently.

If you think that you may come to want to train or work less than full-time in the future, it is worth exploring how easy or hard this could be in different specialties. It can be hard to look ahead at how you might view things in the future. A review by the Institute for Fiscal Studies (IFS) found an inverse relationship between the proportion of women working in the specialties and the number of hours they typically work upon returning after a period of maternity leave. Their review includes a helpful specialty map.[4]

Planning in steps

As you explore, you will notice that some options allow decisions to be made stage by stage. In this sense, Internal Medical Training (IMT) could be a good choice for people who need more time to make up their minds. For the 'Group 2 Specialties' like allergy, dermatology and oncology (for example) the specialties recruit doctors who have followed two years of IMT. The 'Group 1 specialties' such as acute internal medicine, cardiology, and neurology require applicants to follow IMT training for three years. So by following IMT, you would retain the Group 1 and 2 specialties as options.

In Scotland and Northern Ireland, a Broad Based Training is available to those who struggle to choose between general practice, paediatrics, psychiatry, and internal medicine, and who want to progress to one of the specialties at the conclusion of the two-year programme.

Longlisting

It's a good idea to create a longlist of specialties you'd like to consider—a list as long as you wish. Before compiling it, re-read your list of personal criteria—the list that summarizes what you most need from work. The longlist becomes a tool for keeping the information coming to you organized. One reason we suggest taking the trouble to make a longlist is to maximize your chance of engaging in 'slow thinking'. Once you have a longlist, you'll want to delete or strike through some of the specialties as you edge towards your shortlist. It is helpful to keep a fair record of your process—including the specialties you've considered and dismissed—and why.

All this is quite different from the way we normally tackle decisions. Typically we google issues, scan-read whatever is thrown up, rely on our memory, and reach a quick decision. Sometimes we procrastinate, putting off the decision till the last minute.

Consider Jess's longlisting process, discussed in Box 3.1 and Table 3.3.

Shortlisting

The next step is very simple—so simple, it's tempting to skip it altogether. The step is to copy the options that survived into a shortlisting table. Include all the options you want to continue thinking about. If in doubt, review your personal criteria—those that emerged from the self-knowledge exercises in Chapter 2. These can change over time so can be edited at any point.

The layout of the shortlisting table differs from the longlisting table. In the first column, note your personal criteria. The remaining columns are for shortlisting the specialties. To help you move from fast, biased thinking to slower systematic thinking, rate each specialty on each criterion. Use a numerical scale (1 to 5 scale or 1 to 10) just

Box 3.1 **Jess's longlisting**

The variety appearing in Jess's longlist (Table 3.3) may seem implausible. But in our work with doctors, we find that many doctors really do want to consider a great many specialties. Jess preferred the idea of ultimately being hospital-based but she kept General Practice on her longlist as she had got so much out of her student GP attachment. But Jess had felt positively about *most* of her clinical attachments. She knew rather little about the day-to-day duties of a microbiologist, but the science involved in the discipline interested her and brought to mind the more interesting aspects of her intercalated BSc. Jess considered neurology but the specialty didn't make it onto the longlist as Jess recalled not getting on particularly well with neuroanatomy.

Jess longlisted several quite specific options, and wondered what it would be like to take an academic route (see later in the chapter). For Jess, variety was important. But variety isn't necessarily about working with a larger number of body systems or conditions. It can be about having a varied working week. For Jess, the longlisting exercise, which put a structure around the decision, had a motivating effect. But it took a few months of browsing and sifting through endless websites before Jess was able to reduce the list.

Table 3.3 Jess's longlist. You can access a downloadable template of this table online (search for this book's ISBN 9780198884873 at https://academic.oup.com and go to the online appendix at the end of the book. See 'Additional Online Content' for further information).

Specialty	Reason for specialty staying on/coming off
Clinical oncology	Want to work with a variety of conditions
Emergency medicine	Exciting environment (except shifts in training years)
General Practice	Enjoyed GP as a student
Intensive care medicine	Too acute, prefer to work with conscious patients
IMT	IMT route—but to what?—can decide later
Allergy	Academic route, good work-life balance, will it be varied enough?
Dermatology	Academic route, good work-life balance, will it be varied enough?
Infectious diseases & medical microbiology	Academic route, good work-life balance

> ## Box 3.2 **Ruba's shortlisting**
>
> Ruba wanted to ensure she could, if needed, return to work in her home country, Sudan, later in her career. So the specialty would need to be one for which realistic career opportunities existed in Sudan.
>
> The options that eventually made it onto Ruba's shortlist might appear not to have much in common with each other but Ruba's logic was unassailable. By carrying out the shortlisting exercise, Ruba was able to be decisive.
>
> Ruba's longlist was unwieldy but when tested against Ruba's personal criteria, many of the specialties didn't make it onto her shortlist. She wasn't surprised by her ratings but found it upsetting to close off options. On reflection, however, she could see it would be more harmful for her career to keep putting off her decision and the time had come for her to make some decisions about her future.

as a selection panel would. Adding a few words of narrative can make it easier to later recall the thoughts behind the numbers.

Many people, wanting to keep things simple, choose a five point scale. But what if you considered one criterion to be twice as important as the others? This may not be the case but sometimes the setting (hospital or community) or geography *are* more important. You can assign a weight to a criterion by giving it greater value than the others. You could use a 1 to 5 scale for all except one criterion. For that exception, you might use a 1 to 10 scale. Or if it really were more important than the others, but not quite twice as important, you might assign a scale of 1 to 7. To avoid confusion, write down the rating scale you choose for each criterion.

Let us consider a case study, Ruba as an example in Box 3.2. Table 3.4 represents Ruba's shortlist and we continue our discussion in Box 3.3. We will take up Ruba's case study once more in Chapter 4.

Chris's shortlisting

Let us now return to Chris (Box 3.4, see also Table 3.5 and Box 3.5) who was drawn to a career in psychiatry. We last discussed him in relation to his experience log in Chapter 2 and can now consider his shortlisting strategy.

There are strong arguments for taking the numerical ratings seriously. This is, after all, what an interview panel does. But there are also arguments for attending to any narrative you have noted as you bring intuition to bear on the situation. This may seem surprising given that we cautioned against allowing cognitive shortcuts to influence things. But—as we will discuss further in Chapter 5, there's a time and place for intuitive thinking. In a nutshell, the more information you have, the more you can trust intuition. If the shortlist feels like a burden, remember that in shortlisting, you are committing only to investigating the specialties—no more than that.

Table 3.4 Ruba's shortlist. You can access a downloadable template of this table online (search for this book's ISBN 9780198884873 at https://academic.oup.com and go to the online appendix at the end of the book. See 'Additional Online Content' for further information).

Personal criteria	Anaesthetics	Intensive care medicine	Cardiology	General Practice	Chemical pathology	Palliative care
Must be hospital-based for most of time 1 to 5	5 Hospital specialty	5 Hospital +++	5	1	5	4 Hospital or community
Must enable practical procedures to be done 1 to 5	4 Procedures, how much variety?	5 Procedures more varied	5	3.5	1	3 Do happen but not a major part of role
Must be possible to do it less than full time 1 to 5	4 Yes	4 Yes	4 Not sure how easy will be to work LTFT	5	5	5
Work as part of a team 1 to 5	3 Consultant is on own in theatre	4 Yes	3 *Need to check*	2 In theory but in practice?	2.5	5
Must be possible to do it in other countries 1 to 5	5 Can be done in home country, all over world	5 Yes	5	2 Different models of primary care	5	Need to check
Total score 5 to 25	21	23	22	13.5	18.5	18?

> ## Box 3.3 **Ruba's shortlisting continued**
>
> Ruba's explorations started with a visit to the Health Education England (HEE) and royal college websites. She also found a *British Medical Journal (BMJ)* careers article about the work of anaesthetics in theatre, in the labour ward, and in the emergency department and read what had attracted the doctors, now consultants, into the specialty. One had made it their mission to create calm environments, acquiring the skills to handle situations that would previously have been anxiety-provoking. Ruba was glad to read that consultant anaesthetists normally take a day to recover after working through the night. She wondered, 'Is this always true?'
>
> Exploring the competition ratios helped Ruba compare the specialties. Next, she needed to consider the stages of the training. Ruba saw that the Acute Care Common Stem (ACCS) route takes a year longer than the traditional core anaesthetic training. Both paths would be followed by higher specialty training. Would ACCS training *really* broaden her skills? Could following the ACCS path keep options open? She also wondered how flexible the ACCS route might be in reality. Could I go into ACCS having not yet decided between Anaesthetics and Intensive Care Medicine? Some authors seemed to be 'on the fence' on this point.
>
> In her online travels, Ruba came across the Society of Acute Medicine where she read first-hand accounts about the teamwork in cardiology and the consultant cardiologist's leadership role. What Ruba read about the training pathway seemed to confirm what she already knew—that to train, she would follow the IMT 3-year pathway and would then apply to specialty training in cardiology at ST4 level. All of these issues raised questions:
>
> - If I can't make up my mind, is ACCS a good way to decide?
> - What's the team working like in anaesthesia? What about in theatre?
> - What's the on-call like for consultants? In practice is it true that you normally take a day to rest after being on-call?
> - For cardiology, Ruba wanted to know about the new developments in the field; how to get involved in clinical trials.
> - Where, ideally, should she try to train in IMT to maximize her chance of gaining experience in cardiology?

What if I am considering an academic career?

Earlier in the chapter, we met Jess whose longlist included options she wanted to consider as part of an academic training. She'd wondered, 'Would this work well as an academic specialty?' In truth, *any* specialty can lend itself to an academic path, research being the method by which medical knowledge develops across the board.

Many doctors are put off by the idea of research, having devoted so much time to studying, revision, and exams. But some do want to study a subject in depth, to

Box 3.4 Shortlisting and decision hygiene

Though Chris had very nearly made a specialty decision just by following his instinct, he decided to interrogate the decision before making it final. His method involved listing his personal criteria and he selected just three options to weigh up. Chris had considered General Practice as the only alternative to psychiatry but a careful exploration of the specialties revealed an additional option—Rehabilitation Medicine. This was a specialty he had not previously known about. Rehabilitation Medicine seemed to score equally highly on several of his personal criteria, but Chris felt he would need to know far more about the range of conditions typically treated in the specialty. So even though he knew relatively little about the specialty, he had faith in the career planning process and shortlisted the option (Table 3.5). It didn't take much for him to come up with a list of questions that he wanted to investigate (Box 3.5).

Table 3.5 Chris's shortlist

Criteria	Psychiatry	GP	Rehabilitation medicine
Unhurried history taking	5	2 As a student, I have time with patients, but it will be less as a GP	5
Time with relatives	5	1	5
Understand condition in patients' lives	5	4	5 Could be highly rewarding
Working in community some of time	5	5	5
Adult patients	5	3	5
Job security	5	5	5
Total score	30	20	30

contribute to scientific progress and the pool of developing knowledge. It's not necessary to know in advance the area you'd like to study. If you answer yes to some of the following questions, it's worth considering whether following a medical academic path might suit you.

- ◆ Would you like to help patients more broadly through scientific enquiry and by creating new knowledge?

- Would you like to attend and exchange ideas at conferences?
- Would you like to read scientific papers?
- Would you like to participate in a study and eventually carry out your own research?
- Do you feel interested when you hear a good academic speaker present new ideas?
- Do you feel interested in research methods and the different interpretations of results?
- Have you done some hands-on research?
- Are you determined and organized?

If following an academic path interests you, try to attend a conference. Doing so may give you the chance to talk to some of the speakers after their talks as well as to peers. If you're still a student, you may be able to apply for an intercalated BSc or MSc, though for practical and financial reasons, not everybody can do so. At some medical schools, a BMedSci is another type of degree, integrated into some courses, which may offer the chance to try your hand at research. When selecting a project from a range of options, try to select one you genuinely find interesting and would enjoy speaking or writing about.

Though there are well-trodden paths for integrated academic and clinical training (see the websites at the end of the chapter), there is still the need to select a specialty. Wanting to follow an academic route does not take away from this need. But it is possible that by looking into the options for research, an interest in a specialty will 'announce' itself to you.

Box 3.5 **Chris's questions**

Psychiatry

How repetitive does psychiatry get? When you're experienced, does the uniqueness of each patient cease to be interesting? How does the work stay fresh?

GP

What are all the ways of being a GP (with specific populations?) that would allow me to work in more detail with each patient (more time for consultations?)

Rehabilitation medicine

How much psychology/psychiatry is there in rehabilitation medicine? Could it be a specialty to consider if I prefer not to give up my medicine? What does a typical patient encounter look like? What are the sub-specialties like? What do you need to do to keep the work fresh?

Summary

We have considered longlisting and shortlisting as a reasonable way to set out your thoughts in the spirit of decision hygiene. Our experience of working with doctors (and our own experience) is that for most of us, decision hygiene goes against the grain. It would be so much easier if we could only use intuition to make up our minds. Doing so would take considerably less time. But as we have argued, your career decision is one of life's bigger decisions. We chose to illustrate decision hygiene through a consideration of how applicants are selected for jobs—including training posts. It would make little sense for those selectors to make considerable effort to choose wisely while the applicants made *their* choices randomly, devoting little time to the process. So, not only have we borrowed the terminology but we have also borrowed the method—admittedly nothing more complicated than a longlist, a shortlist, and some rating scales.

With the benefit of a shortlist, questions may begin to form themselves in your mind. It is these questions that we will now consider in the next chapter. Even if there are no obvious questions and if the websites or books describe the specialty perfectly, we still suggest going ahead with some investigations. Because websites and books are like shop windows whose purpose is to entice you in. Understandably, those in leadership positions—those in royal college positions, for example—want to draw you into the specialty. With the best of intentions, they are likely to present you with information that is *positively biased.* This is welcoming. But you will also want to make up your own mind, based upon what is by now a strong sense of what *you yourself* are looking for in your future work.

As if this were not enough of a reason, another compelling reason to go ahead with some investigation is that in doing so you are likely to become a stronger applicant. It's a win-win situation.

Additional downloadable content

Downloadable templates to assist you when undertaking the exercises and podcasts voiced by the authors are available online. Search for this book's ISBN (9780198884873) at https://academic.oup.com and go to the online appendix at the end of the book. See 'Additional Online Content' for further information.

References

1. **Campion, M.A., Pursell, E.D., & Brown, B.K.** (1988). Structured interviewing: Raising the psychometric properties of the employment interview. *Pers Psychol.* **41**(1):25–42. https://doi.org/10.1111/j.1744-6570.1988.tb00630.x

2. **Schmidt, F.L., & Hunter, J.E.** (1998). The validity and utility of selection methods in personnel psychology: practical and theoretical implications of 85 years of research findings. *Psychol Bull.* **124**(2):262–274. https://doi.org/10.1037/0033-2909.124.2.262

3. **Spurr, L., Harris, J., & Warwick J.** (2022). *So you want to be a brain surgeon? The essential guide to medical careers* (4th ed.). Oxford University Press.

4. **Kelly, E & Stockton, I.** (2022). *Working patterns of doctors and nurses returning from maternity leave.* Institute for Fiscal Studies. https://ifs.org.uk/articles/working-patterns-doctors-and-nurses-returning-maternity-leave

Further information

British Medical Association (BMA) Specialty Explorer https://www.bma.org.uk/advice-and-support/career-progression/finding-the-right-role/specialty-explorer

Clinical Academic Training and Careers Hub (CATCH) https://www.catch.ac.uk/

NHS Health Careers https://www.healthcareers.nhs.uk/explore-roles/doctors/roles-doctors

The Federation of the Royal Colleges of Physicians of the UK https://thefederation.uk/training/specialties

Chapter 4

Investigating options

In this chapter, we will show you how best to look beyond the attractive shop window of the specialty career materials in order to critically appraise each specialty. We start with the tried and tested methods you already know about—taster days and getting involved in various ways with a specialty. We then move on to the less familiar idea of *informational interviewing*—selecting a person who is in a good position to answer your questions from their own experience. For some, this might not seem like a novel idea, but for others, contemplating such an approach is quite challenging. We discuss some of the reasons why the information interview seems to go against the grain and suggest practical ways to overcome the common barriers.

Tried and tested methods

Taster days

Taster days are well known and much loved, but they can be tricky to organize. That taster days exist at all is an acknowledgement that you need to gain exposure to specialties you might not otherwise come across in foundation—but might actually suit you well. Or perhaps you had some minimal previous exposure to the specialty and now need to know more. It's worth thinking about taster days as far in advance as possible so as to get permission to take time from the ward or department. Attending to them early can increase the chance that the experience can itself form part of your application—as evidence of commitment to the specialty. You should be able to find out about local opportunities through your foundation programme or medical school. It's worth also looking online as some of the royal colleges put on events to showcase their specialties.

Clinical audits and quality improvement projects

Immersing yourself in a subject is a good way to find out whether the subject matter and ways of working could suit you. Those leading quality improvement or audit projects often welcome an extra pair of hands to perform tasks like extracting data from records. A clinical audit can start to feel worthless if the cycle can't be repeated. The same is true for other types of quality improvement project. Too often projects founder because the person leading the project didn't have an enthusiastic band of helpers to complete the work before they rotated away. Being part of such a group could even be quite enjoyable! And the subject matter can then play out in your mind, affording you advantages in applications, interviews, and exams.

Conferences

Conferences can broaden your horizons, bringing different perspectives to complement those gained from formal teaching. You're likely to hear from researchers about the workings of health services around the world. You may hear from inspiring patient experts. You can also get a sense of what people think the future may hold for a particular specialty. Undoubtedly you'll learn new skills and find out about the different roles within the specialty. You may even come away feeling more enthusiastic than you had expected. Even if you don't find the subject riveting, this is in itself valuable information—information you'd rather find out sooner than later. Medical students may feel they won't be welcome or may feel afraid to ask for leave to attend a conference. But the fact that subsidized places, grants, and bursaries are made available suggests that students are welcome attendees.

Research

Most doctors and medical students have huge respect for science. This doesn't necessarily mean all want to be academics, but all doctors need and want to be evidence-based in their practice. Getting involved in research adds to your understanding of how the knowledge base develops (or fails to develop as sometimes happens). Having involvement in research can help you be more confident in explaining research to patients, including the limitations of our knowledge. You might have the chance to create a poster or speak about your part of the project at a meeting or conference. Importantly, you'll gain knowledge of the specialty.

There are many ways to gain access to research opportunities. You might notice a lecturer's contact details at the end of a presentation and take the step of contacting them. This could be refreshing for the lecturer who may be used to lecturing to a sea of people whose interest is at best limited.

Undergraduates may have the opportunity to study a subject during an elective period. Opportunities to study for an intercalated degree exist in most medical schools while those on academic foundation programmes will have built-in research time and supervision.

Lectures and talks

In addition to lectures about conditions, protocols, and types of care, many foundation programmes put on careers days, sometimes featuring talks by specialty trainees about their specialties. Speakers are likely to be those who feel happy with their specialty choice, so you will hear about the positives—another bias, if you like—or a 'shop window' presentation. You might approach the speaker after their talk—or the organizer can put you in touch with them.

Perhaps you feel that the tried and tested methods described here will happen naturally. This can happen. But whether the opportunities arise organically, or whether you seek them out as a deliberate career-planning strategy, it's important to keep a record of the information you uncover. So if you help with a clinical audit, attend a conference, or help produce a poster, make a note of any specialty information that comes up—how things work in the specialty, the kinds of patients, settings, or subject matter, etc.

Informational interviews

The informational interview—in which you gain high quality information by interviewing an informant—is commonplace outside medicine. Within medicine the idea might seem odd if you're working alongside other doctors all day. You might think, 'Surely I already know what they could tell me … ' In the next section, we suggest it's helpful to go ahead and do it anyway, because more information leads to better career decisions. As to how you would gain access to the right person, you could approach them via a third party—someone who does their admin for them or who works in their team. For obvious reasons, you won't want to approach them when they're busy in the resuscitation room. The hope is that they will offer you half an hour in a real or virtual space. Some people are more generous than this.

You already have the skills you need

In Chapter 1 we suggested you already have the skills you need for career-planning. The same applies to interviewing a person about their specialty. Having interviewed countless patients, you'll already know it's helpful to start an interview with open questions then to home in on a particular issue with a closed questions or a clarifying comment. You'll also understand the importance of adopting a systematic approach. When it comes to informational interviewing we cannot emphasize enough the importance of planning the interview in advance. If you leave the conversation to chance, it might take unexpected directions. Your interviewee might tell you why their specialty is the only one worth pursuing—which would be heartening but may not answer your specific questions. If your interviewee knows you, they may attempt to convince you that you're well matched to the specialty. But the purpose of the informational interview is to address the questions *you* want to ask. You could use some of the generic questions in Box 4.1, adding your own questions—questions that occurred to you as you shortlisted the options, based upon your own personal criteria.

We want now to return to consider Ruba (Box 4.2)—how she might approach her informational interview. We met Ruba in Chapter 3 as she weighed up her shortlist of Anaesthetics, Intensive Care Medicine, and Cardiology.

We also meet Chris again, who appeared in Chapters 2 and 3. You'll recall that he had enjoyed the Psychiatry placement in his F2 year. Chris's shortlist included Psychiatry, General Practice and Rehabilitation Medicine.

Tips and tricks

As we've suggested, open questions usually yield higher quality information: interviewees are more likely to illustrate what they say with anecdotes from their personal experience. A useful variation is to ask, 'Can you tell me about … '. For example, 'Can you tell me about what it's like being a Consultant in Intensive Care?'. Closed questions

> ## Box 4.1 **Informational interview questions**
>
> - What gives you greatest job satisfaction?
> - What sorts of things make even the experienced consultants nervous?
> - What counts as success in your specialty?
> - What topics crop up when the consultants are meeting together?
> - What topics (other than funding) crop up between consultants and managers?
> - What (other than funding) frustrates consultants the most?
> - What activities make up a good or bad day?
> - What is night-time on-call like for doctors in training and for consultants?
> - How has your job changed over time?
> - How do you think the job could change in the future?
> - What were the biggest challenges you faced in your career?
> - What research or developments in your specialty do you find most interesting?

can be helpful for clarification, e.g. 'So, most consultants are not directly involved in research?' You might wonder about reading from your notes or note-taking while you're talking. Referring to a written list of questions could give your interviewee a sense that you are guiding the interview. It might even feel refreshing for them that the conversation is one they don't have to be responsible for shaping. Afterwards, you'll want to write down the key points. But writing in the moment could get in the way of rapport-building and may limit what your interviewee will tell you.

One question that sometimes arises is how open you should be about your own issues and concerns. Both Ruba and Chris had issues about which they felt sensitive. Ruba was looking for a specialty that she could later practice in her home country. She didn't feel ready to raise this with anybody, reasoning that she could easily work out the answer for herself. She did, however, want to ask a question about whether following the Acute Care Common Stem (ACCS) training was a good way of keeping her options open. Ruba thought she would probably be more comfortable talking to another trainee. Chris wanted to be careful how he framed his concerns about patients becoming behaviourally disturbed. But he found when he did raise the issue, his interviewee talked frankly about the strengths and weaknesses of the unit in which he worked and about some of the measures being introduced to enhance safety for the staff and patients.

It's possible that your interviewee will be very keen for you to apply to their specialty. Your doing so might compliment the specialty. The social demands of the situation can lead you to say you'll probably apply. But of course most people know that career decisions are complex and personal and nobody is going to later hold you to that comment.

Box 4.2 Two doctors' informational interviewees

In considering the informational interview, Ruba first planned to ask about the range of practical skills trainees develop and how consultants retain their skills. These questions could be asked for each specialty. She could also ask about the new developments in the specialty, about the timetable for a typical day, the rewards and stresses and the on-call.

But some questions occurred to Ruba that were specific to anaesthetics: what it's like to be the only anaesthetist in theatre? How do anaesthetists handle feeling pressured to take a particular course of action? How do anaesthetists know if they are doing okay? Ruba had some questions which she thought might be difficult for an older consultant to answer. She wanted to ask, 'If I can't make up my mind, is ACCS* the best way to decide between ITU and Anaesthetics?' but she wanted to address this question to somebody who had themselves faced that particular issue. Researching ACCS training online, Ruba came across some information about a committee for Acute Care Common Stem training. She followed a link to an ACCS training website and noticed five ACCS trainees who looked approachable. It took quite a bit more googling to find their contact details. To increase her chance of success, Ruba approached an ACCS trainee in her hospital who put her in touch with the ACCS training lead.

Chris was weighing up two issues. He wondered what it might be like working with behaviourally disturbed patients? Would he have the temperament to handle situations that might arise? Would he have—or be able to—develop the skills required? Chris decided to talk to a consultant who had been appointed relatively recently. He deliberately didn't want to talk to a psychiatrist specializing in psychiatric intensive care as he felt they might not understand his concerns. He framed the question as, 'How are psychiatrists trained to deal with behavioural disturbance? How is the team supported after an incident?'

Chris was also interested in rehabilitation medicine but had had no exposure in the specialty. He decided to ask his interviewee to talk him through a typical day and a typical week. He also planned to ask about a memorable patient experience, and about the most and the least rewarding parts of the role. In the event, Chris's interviewee was fully expecting Chris to know nothing about the specialty. The two spoke for a full hour, at the end of which some taster days were offered.

* ACCS (acute care common stem training) is a broad-based training programme that equips trainee doctors with the skills and capabilities required to recognize and undertake initial management of the acutely unwell patient.

Possible barriers to fruitful investigation

Through our work with individuals and groups of doctors, we've become familiar with the barriers doctors face in planning their careers. We briefly discuss some of these here and suggest ways of overcoming such barriers.

Barrier No. 1: Reluctance to bother busy people

It can be hard to ask for busy people's time and because medicine is still very hierarchical, this worry is realistic. But things do change! Most doctors, however senior, are also human. They may enjoy talking about their own experience of their work and career and may want to help others who are considering following in their footsteps. The experience of talking to you *could* be the most rewarding moment of that particular person's day.

To break down the barrier in your own mind, try the following thought experiment: imagine that a family friend asked you to talk to their son or daughter who was considering applying to study medicine. They wanted to know what it's really like. How willing would you be to give them a little time? How much time might you give them if they showed themselves to be highly motivated?

Another way to bust through the barrier is to break the task into manageable steps. You could ask yourself a few questions starting with who, what, why, where, when, and how.

- Who can I interview? Who can help me reach this person? Who may be less helpful?
- What specialties do I want to find out about?
- What do I want to ask?
- Why is this important to me?
- Where will I meet them? (though it will be for them to decide, in-between patients in a busy clinic is not ideal!)
- When does it need to happen?
- How will I broach the subject? How will I explain the method?

Barrier No. 2: Your own time pressure

Time is precious. Both you and your interviewee are likely to be busy. It's too easy for such busyness to be a reason for not doing something important. Oliver Burkeman, journalist and time-management expert, named his recent book *Four Thousand Weeks*[1]—the number of weeks we can expect to live. Burkeman suggests part of procrastinating is convincing ourselves that we need to 'first clear the decks'. This might include answering our emails and doing any number of small tasks. But we must accept that the decks may never be clear as the stream of 'stuff' coming in is never-ending.

A useful antidote, illustrated in Figure 4.1, is to think of filling a container (representing the time you have available) with pebbles and sand (representing the large and small tasks you want to do) without them overflowing. You can quickly see that the task would be accomplished most effectively if the large pebbles were first placed in the container before trickling the sand around them.

It's salutary to consider what makes up the big pebbles as well as the sand in your work and personal life. In your actual job you may have few choices, although, you may be able to identify patterns of procrastination that if tackled, could free up small amounts of time. You may also lament the lack of time to call your own when you're

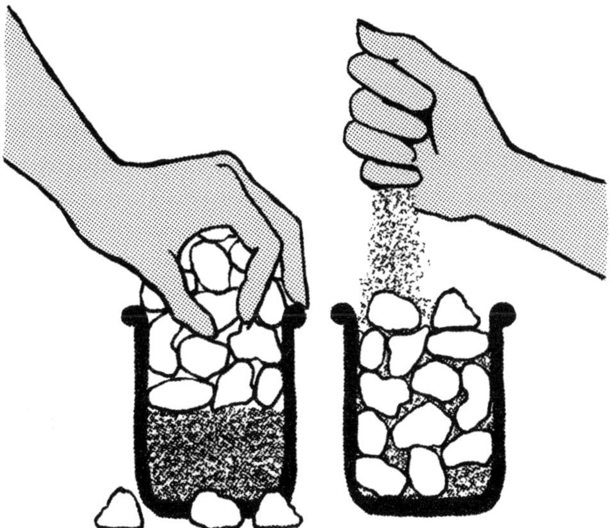

Figure 4.1 Pebble and sand thought experiment.

not at work. Looking specifically at the informational interview, we suggest considering it a larger pebble which might suggest placing it in the vase first, before the items you consider more like sand. This is a long-winded way of saying you need to set aside time for the informational interview.

Pebbles and sand are reminders of a quite different ingredient—grit—fortunately something that most doctors have in abundance. Grit is a construct developed by the psychologist, Angela Duckworth,[2] and is something we demonstrate when we work strenuously towards a challenge. 'Gritty individuals' maintain their effort and interest even when their efforts are thwarted. There is debate about how distinct grit is from conscientiousness, the personality trait. Either way, it is of interest that in surgical trainees,[3,4] grit has been shown to be negatively correlated with burnout. And encouragingly, it's thought that grit is something we *can* develop. To be 'gritty' in relation to a specific goal, it's necessary to give the goal one's full attention and where needed, to be strategic in the way it is carried out. You can be heartened that your perseverance in reading up to this section makes it more likely that you have the grit required to arrange an interview with the right person—and get your unanswered specialty questions answered!

Before we leave this section on time management, we feel compelled to offer one further useful tip from Four Thousand Weeks: instead of having a to-do list, it's helpful to have a list of things you've done. This means ticking off rather than deleting items on your to-do list. Seeing a 'done list' lengthening can be motivating.

Barrier No. 3: The need to show independence

Perhaps as a consequence of the long training and the medical hierarchies, it's easy for doctors in training to feel infantilized. It's not unheard of for colleagues in other health disciplines to speak of 'baby doctors'. So it's understandable to want to prove your independence. Doing so can work well but it's also important to build relationships and to allow yourself to be assisted by other people. There's a strong relationship between building a network and career satisfaction and success.[5,6] It may not *seem* as though asking to meet with a senior doctor to find out about their work could help with network-building but network-building is exactly what it is.

Barrier No. 4: The need for certainty

Living with uncertainty can be difficult, especially if uncertainty in one area has an impact on other aspects of your life. It's tempting to put the issue out of your mind, postpone the decision, or make the decision impulsively without giving it very much time and attention. The developmental psychologist Erik Erikson called this 'Foreclosure'. A phenomenon now recognized by career scholars, foreclosure involves people settling on a career plan without adequately exploring the range of available options.[7,8] For those at risk of either procrastinating or foreclosing a decision it's a good idea to make a project plan with specific times for each action.

Challenging unhelpful thoughts

In the foregoing section, we have tried to convey how easy it is for a host of reasons to come to mind, tempting you to skip the investigation stage. These reasons can, however, be challenged, bringing their influence under your control. They are, after all, only thoughts, and thinking something does not necessarily make it true. In Figure 4.2 we've set out some typical less-than-helpful thoughts together with some possible antidotes: inner conversations sometimes known as positive self-talk.

Some readers will have postponed their career-planning until after their foundation years. They are in good company: it is commonplace to take an F3 year. A report published by Health Education England[9] found that the number of doctors taking an F3 year rose from 17% in 2010 to 65% in 2019—so there's evidence that the majority of doctors don't go straight from foundation into specialty training. But it can be tricky to lose the structure afforded by the training context so it's helpful to think about who you're still in touch who could help—or who could introduce you to someone in the specialty you're interested in.

This chapter's final case study (Box 4.3) illustrates the potential benefits of talking to those who are willing to share their experience.

Christina's case illustrates that the 'investigation stage' is sometimes more than an investigation because the time you spend talking with more senior doctors can make a small but significant contribution to your professional network. We'll come back to network-building in future chapters, as it's such an important topic.

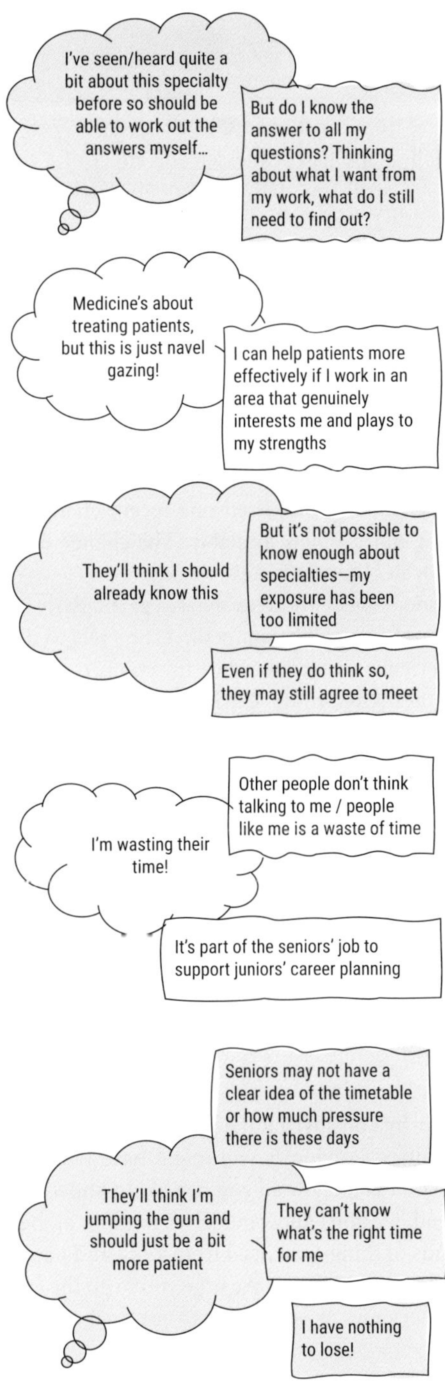

Figure 4.2 Less-than-helpful thoughts and positive self-talk.

> ### Box 4.3 **Asking questions**
>
> Christina had at one time considered Obstetrics and Gynaecology (O&G) but had been put off when she had witnessed the effect of a maternal death on a team. She had also felt 'semi-traumatized' through watching a popular TV drama featuring the specialty. Other options which Christina had had on her short-list were Gastro-enterology and Interventional Radiology. Christina thought of Surgery as male dominated, though she recognized that Obstetrics is more evenly split between the genders.
>
> Because of the strength of her feelings, Christina knew she needed to take stock. She decided to talk to a female O&G consultant and was able to make contact with one through the Royal College. After exchanging emails, the two met online. Christina asked the consultant what it had been like to train, what being a consultant was like, and how O&G consultants are able to gain support when things go wrong. They discussed one recent change: that psychological support is becoming more widely available. The change had been campaigned for by midwife advocates, benefitting everybody.
>
> Christina mentioned one of the areas she was particularly interested in – infertility, which she knew to be highly competitive. She received some useful advice about gaining experience that could have future currency and was advised to consider taking an academic route. Christina had not properly considered the option before, assuming doing so would not be compatible with having a family. They talked about less-than-full time options. 'It is not a race' were the words that hung in Christina's ears as she clicked on 'leave meeting'.
>
> That consultant was close to retirement so had suggested Christina spend time with an ST7 training in fertility. She mentioned a couple of names and electronically introduced Christina to each of them a few days later. The whole experience was a confidence-boosting one which inspired Christina to sign up to a mentoring scheme, and later to apply to train in the specialty.

Summary

We started this chapter by considering the various different ways of answering your questions about specialties. Previously you might have thought you didn't have any particular questions—that you knew all you needed to know. Sometimes, if questions aren't really encouraged, we don't allow ourselves to think of them. But once you have thought about the kinds of things you need from work and have started to explore the options, questions will inevitably arise. We urge you to go the extra mile and carry out some informational interviews in order to put your final career decision onto a solid footing.

References

1. **Burkeman, O.** (2021). *Four thousand hours.* UK Penguin, Random House.
2. **Duckworth, A.L., Peterson, C., … & Kelly, D.R.** (2007). Grit: perseverance and passion for long-term goals. *J Pers Soc Psychol.* **92**(6):1087. https://doi.org/10.1037/0022-3514.92.6.1087
3. **Salles, A., Cohen, G.L., & Mueller, C.M.** (2014). The relationship between grit and resident well-being. *Am J Surg.* **207**(2):251–254. DOI:10.1016/j.amjsurg.2013.09.006
4. **Hewitt, D.B., Chung, J.W., … & Bilimoria, K.Y.** (2021). National evaluation of surgical resident grit and the association with wellness outcomes. *JAMA Surg.* **156**(9):856–863. DOI:10.1001/jamasurg.2021.2378
5. **Wolff, H.G., & Moser, K.** (2009). Effects of networking on career success: a longitudinal study. *J Appl Psychol.* **94**(1):196. https://doi.org/10.1037/a0013350
6. **Ng, T.W., & Feldman, D.C.** (2014). Subjective career success: a meta-analytic review. *J Vocat Behav.* **85**(2):169–179. https://doi.org/10.1016/j.jvb.2014.06.001
7. **Borges, N.J., Navarro, A.M., & Grover, A.C.** (2012). Women physicians: choosing a career in academic medicine. *Acad Med.* **87**(1):105–114. DOI: 10.1097/ACM.0b013e31823ab4a8
8. **Polenova, E., Vedral, A., … & Zinn, L.** (2018). Emerging between two worlds: A longitudinal study of career identity of students from Asian American immigrant families. *Emerg Adulthood.* **6**(1):53–65. https://doi.org/10.1177/2167696817696430
9. **Royal College of Physicians & NHS England.** (2022). *The F3 Phenomenon: Exploring a new norm and its implications.* https://www.hee.nhs.uk/sites/default/files/documents/F3_Phenomenon_Final.pdf

Further reading

Duckworth, A. (2017). *Grit: Why passion and resilience are the secrets to success.* Vermillion.

Chapter 5

The decision

Crunch time: we have now arrived at the actual decision. This is rarely a binary choice as career decisions typically break down further into smaller decisions. With our clinical practice analogy, an initial decision about a patient's diagnosis might move seamlessly into a decision about the type or stage of the condition. This is the case also with career decisions. The first career decision might be a specialty choice. Other decisions flow from this one, such as whether to pursue an academic pathway or to train part-time. In this sense career planning is more of a process than an event.

In this chapter we will discuss some common aspects of decision-making and we offer some tools to facilitate decision hygiene. But we start by briefly revisiting human resource practices to illustrate an important key principle that we suggest keeping in mind.

Back-up options

If you are on the receiving end of a selection panel, you may surmise that the panel will not only select a favourite applicant (hopefully based on their knowledge, skills and experience) but also, knowing that the favourite candidate may well receive other offers, the panel will, if they can, select one or more back-up candidate. Earlier in the book we suggested it's a two way street as every time somebody applies for a job, both the recruiter and the applicant are making choices. In other words, both sides are selecting, so you can take a leaf out of the recruiter's book. Keeping your own shortlist active for a while may not appeal as it necessitates tolerating uncertainty. But doing so may provide you with some vital back-up options.

Why have back-up options?

Fredkin's paradox is a succinct argument in favour of retaining back-up options. Edward Fredkin, a Professor of Robotics at Carnegie Mellon University, devoted much of his career to understanding the connections between physics and the digital sciences. Fredkin's paradox (Box 5.1) states, rather poetically, that we can waste a lot of time agonizing between equally attractive options.

Fredkin's paradox might seem counter to the approach we encouraged in our earlier chapters—taking time to review your interests and talents and what you most need from your work, then exploring the options carefully, before making a choice. But of course the reason for doing so was not to identify 'the one' but '*the ones*', which might meet your needs.

> ## Box 5.1 **Fredkin's paradox**
>
> "The more equally attractive two alternatives seem, the harder it can be to choose between them—no matter that, to the same degree, the choice can only matter less."

In deciding how many back-up options to keep, a helpful guide is the degree of competition expected. In the UK, this data is published in the form of Competition Ratios—a metric that tells us the number of people who apply for each specialty training vacancy. Imagine you were drawn to a specialty in which 20 people applied for each post. In that scenario, you would be wise to retain a back-up option. Or more than one if your back-up option also had a high competition ratio.

Duration of training

Looking ahead at training in a specialty, it also seems sensible to consider how long the training will take. The three-year training for general practice is relatively short. Other trainings might take 7 or 8 years, full-time, and considerably longer if you train less-than-full-time, sub-specialize, or follow an academic route. It makes sense to think through what a very lengthy training might feel like. For some people, being out-of-sync with peers to continue training and take exams as a mature adult will feel fine. For others it may feel problematic. Conversely, we have occasionally observed that some doctors, who came to feel unhappy with general practice had initially chosen the specialty for its shorter training—rather than out of an inherent interest in the challenges and rewards of working in primary care. It's wiser, therefore, to consider what the specialty itself has to offer—what the job involves doing, and how well this maps on to your individual job needs.

Intuition gets a look-in!

Notwithstanding the structured approach we have encouraged, you'll recall that Decision Hygiene encourages the use of intuition *once all the data is in*. We see this in practice in our work with doctors: once the groundwork has been done the career decision can sometimes seem to make itself. You might be familiar with the story, possibly apocryphal, of the discovery of the molecular ring structure of benzene by Kekulé, who is said to have day-dreamed a snake biting its tail. The novel *Frankenstein* and the Beatles song *Yesterday* are said to have come to their respective creators Mary Shelley and Paul McCartney in their sleep. They exemplify the power of non-conscious thinking.

Applying intuition or non-conscious thinking to the task of decision-making, recall the analogy of the elephant and the rider in which the decision-maker is the elephant (non-conscious thinking) rather than the rider. So a decision can occur in a moment of reverie: while jogging, walking, taking a shower, or sleeping. Or a decision can form itself more gradually. However it happens, it's important to interrogate it systematically in a final validating stage.

Options appraisals

An options appraisal is really just a list of pros and cons applied to one or more options—a way of injecting some objectivity into the checking process. Each option can be scored or ranked. Another method is to write a note against each option. Using numerical scores doesn't necessarily mean you have to choose the highest scoring option. Seeing the scores can bring about a sense of misgiving. If so, it's then important to 'interrogate' your gut feeling. What do you find yourself thinking about the option? It may be something you have not yet factored in but which turns out to be critically important to you.

An options appraisal can be helpful for various kinds of difficult decision, not just career planning—from choosing between different service delivery models to decisions closer to home (Figure 5.1).

How does all this work in practice? In Boxes 5.2 and 5.3 we consider how an options appraisal (Table 5.1) might aid a career decision.

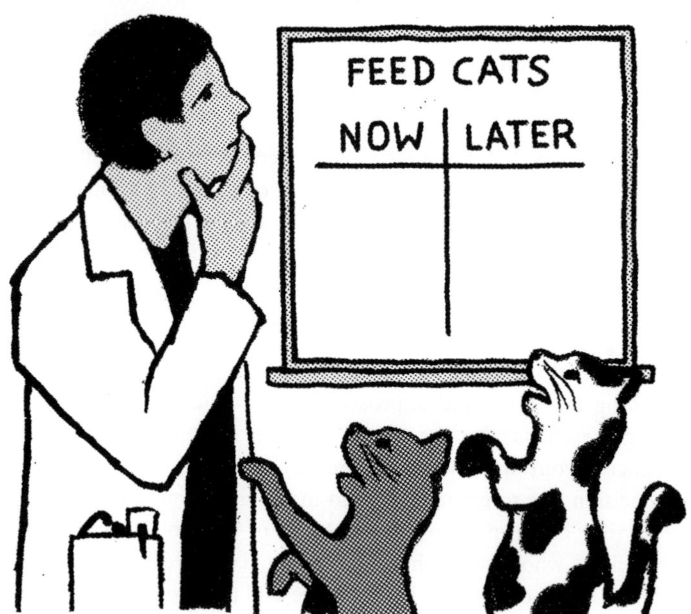

Figure 5.1 To feed or not to feed?

Box 5.2 **An interesting idea**

Tom's foundation programme was surgically oriented. He developed some good experience for an application to core surgical training. He also considered general practice with a view to being a GP with a special interest in orthopaedics. After his foundation year (FY) posts, Tom took an F3 year, working in an emergency department. Tom met an inspiring event doctor who invited him to go along as an observer to a sports tournament. Tom came away from the day feeling more excited about work than usual. Being sociable and enjoying teamwork, Tom enjoyed working in hospitals. He was a keen sportsman, having played football and cricket at quite a high level. More recently, he'd been into hill running and snowboarding (when he had the chance). It dawned on Tom that he could look into a career as a GP with a special interest in sports injury. To work as a sports medicine physician seemed too good to be true, knowing how few training places were available, but a GP with a special interest seemed more realistic. Previously, he had wanted to be hospital-based but his growing interest in sports medicine made him reconsider. He now wondered what working in a community setting might be like once he had established some routines and networks. Putting the arguments for and against the options in a table helped Tom handle the uncertainty. It also gave him the confidence to broach the subject with his family and husband.

Table 5.1 Tom's options appraisal

	For	Against	Score	Reflection
Sports medicine	Working in non-medical environments Patients well, competitive Psychological issues	Extreme competition May be seen as less serious Less variety	5	If I don't like it, can move to GP with special interest
Orthopaedic surgery	Operating will be interesting, new developments likely Hospital-based	Competitive Hospital career may lose its appeal later	4	Could do core training then apply to Sport and Exercise (S&E) OR Orthopaedics OR both
Emergency medicine	Varied Hospital-based	Rotas stressful Hospital career may lose its appeal later	3	Can do ED then try for S&E with Orthopaedics as back-up
GP	More varied, more autonomy, can develop a special interest	I could burn out	4	Good base for developing interests

> ## Box 5.3 **With the benefit of an options appraisal**
>
> Finding himself writing the words, 'Extreme competition' in the 'against' column had a motivating effect on Tom. He formed a game plan: to apply for core surgical training, to get some orthopaedics experience. This could then give him a choice of continuing in Orthopaedics, trying for Sport and Exercise medicine, or re-training as a GP.
>
> Tom realized this could be a long-winded way to become a GP but he wondered if a three-year training might for him feel quite short. He thought he could be very fulfilled as a GP with a special interest in sports medicine and started to wonder whether he could find a practice that served a university where a lot of sport was played. Tom had sleepless nights going through the choices, realizing he had many potentially fulfilling options.

An imaginary future

Tom was able to look into and anticipate how he might feel in the future. Some people enjoy planning; for them, planning the journey is part of its enjoyment and Tom was in that category. But what if you are not, and find planning hard?

In the romantic comedy *Sliding Doors* Gwyneth Paltrow's character Helen is fired. As Helen, clutching her bag of personal effects, takes a train home, we see her meet the man of her dreams. The film cuts to an alternate version of events, the train doors sliding closed so Helen doesn't meet this man. Life isn't like the movies. We rarely get to experience both stories—but this doesn't stop us imagining them.

The following exercises can help you imagine your future self. Holding up the options, you can gauge your inner elephant's response. We don't mean to imply that you can predict the future but it can be a useful exercise, nonetheless.

Exercise: Fast-forward 10 years

Picture yourself, with your actual personality (and with a few more grey hairs), ten years from now. Now bring to mind the specialty you're currently considering. Imagine you trained in that specialty and are now quite a few years post-CCT. Write down how you might spend your time day-to-day. What might this feel like? How might you tend to speak about what you do to others?

One day a colleague asks you to look after a stand at a careers fair. You agree to do it. On the day, a steady stream of students and doctors ask you about your specialty.

- What gives you job satisfaction?
- What sorts of things worry you?
- What's a typical day like?
- What does a bad day look like?

- What's life like when you're not working?
- What keeps you awake at night?

These questions might seem oddly familiar, being similar to those we suggested for informational interviews (Chapter 4). This time, however, it's you who's answering them.

The point of the exercise is to picture yourself in this hypothetical specialty and you could repeat the process for different specialties. You may find your elephant's intuition kicking in, making one specialty feel more natural for you than some of the others. You could interrogate this intuition: what exactly is it that your elephant is responding to?

Exercise: Fast-forward to retirement

Picture yourself many years from now. You've had a long and successful career. Finally, you decided to retire. Your family threw a party for you and playfully presented you with a lifetime achievement award. They recruited a friend to speak about you—and you yourself said a few words.

- What might your friends say about you as a person and what had motivated you?
- What was your habitual way of working?
- What might be said about your home life?
- Has anything about the way you worked influenced younger doctors in their careers?
- How did you describe yourself and your relationship to your work?

Do these imagined thoughts have any implications for the specialties you are currently weighing up? Do you notice any kind of reaction on the part of your inner elephant?

Taking your misgivings seriously

You will by now realize that your inner elephant is much more straightforward in its likes, dislikes, and fears than your rider. Riders can of course disregard any misgivings the elephant may have. But now you have reached the stage of career planning in which you need to give serious consideration to any misgivings.

You'll recall that we suggested that the exercises in Chapter 2 be solitary activities. The time has come for you to talk about the options you're considering with those people most important to you and who know you well. As you speak to others, try to notice what you yourself are saying. Your true feelings may 'out' themselves in what you find yourself saying (or hesitating to say). If you find yourself saying, 'If I don't like it, I can always change', you could wonder what's stopping you from changing your plan right away.

Possible barriers to making a decision

In this chapter so far, we've allowed intuition to take on a greater role in the making and validating of the decision. We've considered that the decision might not be a simple binary one and that back-up plans are often important. We now want to consider three possible barriers each with the potential to throw you off course.

Barrier No. 1: The need to please others

Historically, it was quite common for people to engage in work similar to that of their families—and that included medicine.[1] Medicine was and is still seen as a secure profession: there will, it is reasoned, always be a need for doctors. You may even have a sense that a family member has a particular specialty in mind for you. Perhaps they are influenced by having followed a particular path themselves or they know you well and feel that a particular specialty would suit you. Now through discussing your plans, you'll be able to reality-check your assumptions about what key people in your life are thinking. It may be interesting to hear what your significant others make of your plans, and particularly important if they will themselves be affected. So there are compelling reasons to talk about the plans you're making and your underlying reasoning. A case study (Box 5.4) exemplifies this.

George's inner dialogue could have been similar to that in Figure 5.2.

Barrier No. 2: Continuation bias

Continuation bias, also known as the Sunk Cost Fallacy, is one of the cognitive shortcuts alluded to in Chapter 1. Experimental psychology shows that when we have a forced choice between holding onto something we had earlier gained or gaining something greater in the future, we are generally biased in favour of safeguarding the smaller gain we have already made. The tendency is accentuated if there is a tangible disadvantage to changing but it can occur even in the absence of a disadvantage other than the discomfort of switching. We seem to reason, 'As I've put so much time and effort into my training, I need to stick with the plan'.

So how can we offset this tendency? Tools like options appraisals and future-oriented exercises may help. It's also useful to remember that medicine is full of transferable skills. Skills you developed in one training setting can often be used in another. An audit in a fracture clinic might have a lot in common with one in an eye clinic. An experience you had in one part of your career can be unexpectedly helpful later on. You may find it helpful to try an inner dialogue, identifying and challenging the less-than-helpful thoughts about continuity (Figure 5.3).

Barrier No. 3: Perfectionism

Perfectionism, the personality trait in which we strive for flawless performance, is common among doctors. It's likely that perfectionistic people self-select *and* are selected into the profession. And that the culture of medicine then further accentuates this trait in doctors.[2,3] But perfectionism may not reliably improve our performance.[4] This principle can also apply to doctors' career decision-making. Doctors who procrastinate in their career decision-making sometimes tell us that no option seemed right, so they waited for too long for the perfect option to show itself. The doctor in our case study in Box 5.5 did manage to break out of procrastination but it took some time.

Box 5.4 **I didn't want you to be disappointed**

George's parents are both GPs. He is the only one of his siblings to have become a doctor. Throughout his career George had expressed an interest in oncology and he now had sufficient experience for a strong application. While working with cancer patients and subsequently in his respiratory placement, George worked closely with an exemplary palliative care team and came to think of the palliative care consultant as a role model.

George arranged a taster week with the palliative care team. He was struck by the team dynamic. The team seemed not to be 'organized' by the principle of buying time for the patient at all costs but instead attended empathically to quality of life issues. George was also interested in the transparent nature of the conversations within the team, with patients and families, and the way in which decisions about end-of-life care were integral to the work and didn't feel like optional add-ons, as they had in other specialties.

George 'knew' his parents would be disappointed as they had always seemed so excited by his oncology plan. But when he raised his change of plan with them, they were keen to hear all about it. It emerged that what they'd been excited about was not so much the specifics of the plan, but that George *had a plan that excited him.* They both had huge respect for both oncology and palliative care and his mother went on to describe how she was reviewing end-of-life prescribing in her GP practice.

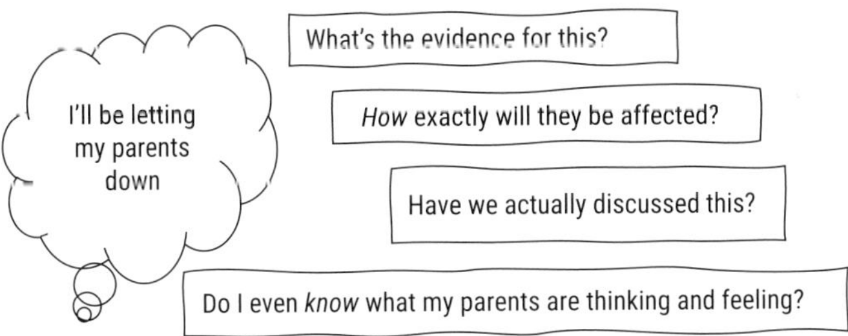

Figure 5.2 A classic worry.

We tend to think of perfectionism as part of our personality so assume it is unchangeable. But how we think, feel, and behave can still be brought under our control. Noticing perfectionism at work can be very freeing. Taking some time out can help put some perspective on a situation. It doesn't need to be a whole year: a week or two could be sufficient. Alternatively, talking to a different person to those you normally talk to could also help you challenge unhelpful ideas.

Many other barriers may thwart your decision-making. Some decision points are challenging in a way particular to that specific decision. It can be painful to let go of an

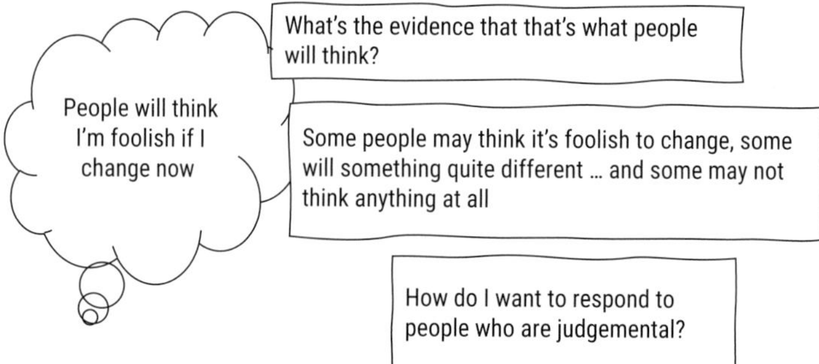

Figure 5.3 Ideas about continuity.

option that had previously seemed so promising. And it can be tricky to live with the uncertainty of maintaining a range of options for a period sufficient to allow a front-runner to emerge. But for most people, following the structure outlined in this book enables them to get to a point where they feel comfortable making a decision.

Box 5.5 **Having doubts and taking time**

Dorothy put her all into her work. As a highly empathic individual, she was always the one to offer to help out and she couldn't bear to see a colleague struggle to fill rota gaps. Instead, she'd always offer to fill the gap herself.

Because Dorothy hadn't a clue what to do, she decided to take a year out to work in Australia and to travel in Southeast Asia. She had found it easiest to get work in an emergency department. Even though this had not been Dorothy's first choice specialty, she got a tremendous amount out the year. On returning to the UK, Dorothy picked up shifts in the emergency department (ED). With no longer-term career plan, she reconciled herself to taking an F4 year.

It was surprising for Dorothy to find herself so stuck having performed really well in F1 and F2. One problem was that she could see both the positives and the negatives of each option she considered. She had many options on her short-list including obstetrics and gynaecology (O&G), dermatology, renal medicine, endocrinology, and psychiatry. Dorothy began to realize that her perfectionism (i.e. needing to find the perfect specialty) led to prevarication.

But the extra time afforded by 'F4' year was invaluable. It allowed Dorothy to be systematic—in the ways we suggest in this book. She developed a routine of 'cold calling' registrars to ask them how she might set up an observational placement. There were hurdles to overcome: Dorothy disliked asking for favours, much preferring giving to receiving, but as Dorothy was known to everybody (and was recognized as being particularly obliging), she eventually realized that others *wanted* to help her.

Summary

In this chapter we have allowed intuition to take its rightful place but have observed that this might not necessarily make decision-making feel any easier. For this reason, we continue to advocate for structure. Some of us have to keep a number of irons in the fire for longer than others. At the same time many of us have perfectionistic traits, so will benefit from a logical approach to career planning.

However easy or hard it is to arrive at a career decision, once you have done so, it's worth acknowledging or even celebrating it as a landmark in your journey. There is still plenty to do—and the ongoing journey will throw up many further decisions. But making a decision is undoubtedly an important step forward.

References

1. **School of Life** (2017). *A job to love.* The School of Life Press.
2. **Firth-Cozens, J.** (1998). Individual and organizational predictors of depression in general practitioners. *Br J Gen Pract.* **48**(435):1647–1651.
3. **Gautam, M.** (2000). Depression and anxiety. In: Goldman L.S., Myers, M., & Dickstein L.J., eds. The handbook of physician health. American Medical Association; 80–94.
4. **Harari, D., Swider, B.W., ... & Breidenthal, A. P.** (2018). Is perfect good? A meta-analysis of perfectionism in the workplace. *J Appl Psychol.* **103**(10):1121. https://doi.org/10.1037/apl0000324

Chapter 6

Applying for a position

Feeling ready to apply for training posts is an achievement even if it may rattle your nerves. One challenge is that the application process can throw up further decisions, making the decision-making feel never-ending. In this chapter we will discuss these 'secondary' decisions as well as the application process itself.

An approach we suggest is to see the game-like qualities in the application process. Our intention is not to be flippant but to recognize the complexity of the situation. In games, there are rules to be discovered. Strategies can be taken to make winning more likely. One of the characteristics of 'the game' that frustrates UK doctors is that the rules change frequently. While we discuss some of the rules prevailing at the time of writing, we know that they are likely to may be replaced with new rules. We therefore also discuss some of the general principles as well as some tips and tricks. We cover competition ratios, whether to apply to a training rotation at all, and whether to apply for one or multiple specialties. Finally there can be different routes each with advantages and disadvantages. The complexity of 'the game' can cause some to hesitate to engage. Our hope is that if doing so will meet your needs, you'll feel encouraged to proceed.

Principle 1: Not all information is equal

With games, it's common for different players to have their own version of the rules. For this, though, the game that sets up your career, we suggest sourcing the rules from the most up-to-date and reliable source. That is not to say that intelligence from friends, bloggers, vloggers, and commercial organizations has no place. There is some excellent and informative content to be found but it's also essential to check the facts with the 'official' websites.

Principle 2: Time is fickle

Having sat numerous exams, most doctors want to know the timetable for application forms going live and submission deadlines. Knowing how much time you have is important. Even with this knowledge, most of us still overestimate how much we can accomplish in a given time. As we fall prey to 'optimism bias', discussed in Box 6.1, we find out that time is not our friend!

In a sober 'how-to' piece, Health Education England reported on the Specialty Trainee applications that were received by the Oriel system in 2015.[2] The average time applicants took to complete their application was 11 days. A sizeable minority (8.4%) had started their application just 24 hours or less before the deadline. Of these, only 6% received a training offer, compared with 58% of all applicants. The offer rate decreased to 3% for those applying in just 60 minutes from start to finish.

> ## Box 6.1 **Optimism bias**
>
> Optimism bias is the difference between a person's expectation and the outcome that follows. Experimental studies show that we are selective in how we attend to incoming information that contradicts our expectations. We respond preferentially to information suggesting things will be better than we expect. By comparison, we tend to neglect information suggesting things will be less good. This occurs even for those very expert in their fields—sometimes causing doctors to overestimate the likely benefits of a particular treatment.[1]
>
> It is quite widely known that individuals who become depressed lose their optimism bias, and when depression is severe, optimism bias is replaced with pessimism bias. There are advantages to being optimistically biased—and there are risks. At a societal level, our tendency towards a lack of preparedness for natural disasters may be attributable to optimism bias—something that we saw all too clearly at the time of the COVID-19 pandemic.

It makes sense to break the process down into stages. Even a simple task like emailing your referees can take longer than expected. Some referees respond quickly, while others are busy or slow. The same is true for the process of uploading supporting evidence. With this in mind, it's worth guessing how long a stage will take, then making an extra time allowance to correct for optimism bias.

There are only 24 hours in the day, and many of these are already taken up with working, sleeping, and eating. As Oliver Burkeman reminds us in his eponymous time management book, we can expect to live for an average of *Four Thousand Weeks*.[3] Burkeman logically suggests that if time is in short supply, *something* needs to give, if only temporarily. One solution is to plan over a longer period, allowing you to allocate smaller chunks of time which work cumulatively. Another advantage to starting early is that you will notice the gaps in your experience in time to remedy them. Our case study in Box 6.2 demonstrates that by starting early, you may better learn the rules of the game.

But it's not always possible to plan ahead. The world can challenge us, throwing up unexpected opportunities with tough deadlines. No matter how much or how little time you have, it's helpful to have an organized plan of attack and a structured approach to the last checks before clicking on 'submit'. This could include asking a trusted friend or family-member to read your application checking for typos.

It's unlikely most people will take to learning the rules of the game with quite such alacrity as Alex who had an off-the-scale level of self-efficacy. So—what exactly is self-efficacy and how can it be developed? Self-efficacy is not unlike efficacy in medicine (which sometimes must be distinguished from effectiveness). There are distinctions to be made in psychology too—as we explain in Box 6.3.

We can begin to think of self-efficacy as a most important set of beliefs impacting our behaviour and our careers. Even if we can't influence our cultural, education, and work environments, there may still be things we can do to develop our self-efficacy.

Box 6.2 **Taking the game to the next level**

Alex was the kind of person who appeared not to worry about the future. She opted for IMT to give her as much choice as possible and was busily preparing for a Group 2 specialty which would mean a specialty training application after just two years.

Alex had friends a little further ahead than she was. She'd heard them complain bitterly while stressing about getting applications done, particularly when system-changes had occurred and she learnt a lot just by listening to what other people were going through. From an early stage, Alex treated the Oriel system as if it were a maze and she a laboratory rat exploring it. She made the rat run the maze in various different ways—starting applications that she had no intention of submitting, just to see how the system worked and what sort of evidence she would need to upload as part of the process. When the system's bots generated messages reminding her to complete an application, Alex would joke that she was perverting the statistics, or that her probity could be called into question. Such an idea might have unnerved some people but the process gave Alex a very practical level of information.

When it came to Alex's actual application, engaging with the system from an informed position meant that she already had documents scanned, filed, and formatted and could ask her seniors to be her referees in good time. As Alex began to apply for specialty training (ST) posts in haematology, medical microbiology, and nuclear medicine, she already knew the rules of the game.

Consider:

- that your role models are the people who represent the sort of person you hope to be. Seeing a role model succeed is likely to increase your own career self-efficacy. Who are your most important role models? How could you increase your exposure to their positive influence?

- Could you talk to peers or seniors? Could someone you ordinarily interact with be a helpful influence? Or could you approach a potential role model you don't yet know well?

- Would you ask for career support or mentoring? A mentor may be able to help you identify hurdles and gain confidence to overcome them.

- Considering the 'rules of the game' discussed earlier. What are the next challenges in the game for you? What does your timetable look like?

Competition ratios

Medical students and doctors will have achieved their current status through a highly competitive selection processes. The fact of having already 'got in' can, however, create a blind spot to the ongoing competition. We therefore suggest checking out the

Box 6.3 **Self-efficacy and career self-efficacy**

First proposed by one of the psychology greats, Albert Bandura,[4] *self-efficacy* is a person's *belief* in their own ability to accomplish things. This is not necessarily the same as the person's *actual* efficacy. Our self-efficacy can develop in four ways. Firstly, we learn through our experience of working towards and accomplishing our goals. Secondly, we learn by observing others as they work towards and accomplish their goals. In our case study, this worked for Alex who took a keen interest in other people's applications. A third influence is social persuasion—if someone tells you you're fully competent and 'should go for it'. Fourthly we make inferences about our abilities by perceiving and interpreting our physiological and emotional states.

Self-efficacy can be applied to our career-related behaviour, with so-called *career self-efficacy* referring to people's beliefs about the efficacy of their behaviour in relation to progressing their career choices.[5]

In a US study with biomedical students, as well as varying with seniority, those lower in self-efficacy were more likely to be female members of under-represented ethnic groups. These students were less confident in their ability to progress to research positions. Family and cultural expectations are likely to be important, possibly interacting with factors in the learning environment. The authors wondered if the students' self-efficacy might benefit from diverse role models being visible and mentoring support being made available.[6]

In other studies in which students reported on their job-searching behaviour, positive relationships were shown between career self-efficacy, the intensity of the job-searching, the number of interview offers received and the number of job offers received—ultimately affecting the students' chances of being employed.[7–9]

published competition ratios for the specialties you are considering. A competition ratio is the number of people who applied for each advertised post.

Table 6.1 shows several years' competition ratios for entering four specialties at CT1 or ST1 level: obstetrics and gynaecology; clinical radiology; anaesthetics; and cardiothoracic surgery. For each, the overall trajectory has been towards greater competition.

But competition ratios are blunt instruments. Many details of the recruitment process do not inform the ratio. In particular:

- Ratios differ in different geographical areas.
- The published data can lead you to assume each person applies for one post. But some doctors make multiple applications, elevating the competition ratios.
- Competition ratios are a function of all the applications received including those made the day before the deadline and those that were dashed off in an hour—which,

Table 6.1 Competition ratios for four specialties

	Obstetrics & Gynaecology	Clinical Radiology	Anaesthetics	Cardiothoracic Surgery
2014	2.4	3.5	2.1	10
2016	2.0	4.3	2.1	10
2018	1.9	3.8	2.5	8
2020	2.6	4.2	2.6	9.9
2022	3.7	6.2	4.2	19.6
2023	4.3	8.8	4.8	27

Data from https://www.specialty-applications.co.uk/competition-ratios/

as we have seen, are unlikely to yield an offer. If you apply in a timelier way, your chance may be greater than the ratio suggests.

- It's hard to compare competition ratios for specialties with larger numbers of applicants against smaller specialties for which the competition ratios are more variable.
- With 'uncoupled' training (core training, CT, and higher specialist training, ST) each stage has its own selection process and associated competition ratio.
- It is also worth looking into the number of consultant posts in the specialties, particularly if in the long term you hope to work in a particular geographic area.

Even taking all of these points into account, competition ratios can still be dispiriting. You might wonder what you can do to increase your chance of success. We suggest choosing between two different 'game plans'.

Game Plan A: Apply for the training post you want

In recent years, two-thirds of applicants made just one application per 'round'.[2,10] By taking this approach, the applicants will have inadvertently reduced their chance of being offered a training place. Many would need to re-apply later, following a non-training path in the interim. Such a path could involve travelling and working abroad or finding a clinical fellowship. Some doctors choose to work flexibly, through a staff bank. Doing one of these appeals to those wanting a break from training to 're-charge their batteries'.

The case study in Box 6.4, Anil, is an example of a doctor using Game Plan A.

For Anil, the decision was straightforward, and his 'F3 year' allowed him to hone his experience over the crucial six month period. For some this might take a year or more. If longer, it is important not to accumulate so much non-training experience in a specialty that you become ineligible to apply for a training post in that specialty. Several

> ### Box 6.4 **Collecting the best 'hand' you can**
>
> Determined to train in London, Anil was not deterred by not being offered a core medical training (equivalent to IMT training) at his first application. Anil put his energy into finding a post that would provide the level of training and supervision he needed. Though tempted by ad hoc locum work and a more relaxed schedule, Anil decided this would be a risky strategy for him.
>
> Anil found a clinical fellowship in metabolic medicine and endocrinology at a London teaching hospital. He received excellent supervision, and with the encouragement of his seniors, took every opportunity to teach and get involved in research. Anil started studying for his MRCP. It seemed strange to be working so hard in this, his 'F3 year' when many friends were taking it easy, some travelling. But Anil had already had a taste of travel prior to starting at medical school and wanted to use the time to focus on getting an IMT post. Anil's choice of strategy paid off. By the next round of applications, he had a solid support network. Several doctors further along in their careers were willing to read through Anil's application, pointing out some achievements that he'd overlooked. Including these helped him gain him more points.
>
> Anil excelled at his interview, ranking sufficiently highly to be offered one of his training choices. Anil is now a Consultant in Diabetes and Endocrinology at two London hospitals. Wherever possible he encourages his colleagues to create clinical fellowships, knowing from his first-hand experience that these posts provide great value, not only for the hospital, but also for the 'F3' doctors.

specialties set an upper limit on how much experience candidates can have at the start of their training so it is worth checking the person specifications carefully.

Game Plan B: Apply for more than one specialty

Game Plan B, illustrated with a case study in Box 6.5, involves applying for a number of training posts simultaneously.

Earlier in the book we suggested that for many of us, there may be more than one career path that would suit us well. And the centralized application system welcomes applicants making multiple specialty applications. It's often, therefore, a question of looking at what the specialties have in common rather than their differences. Confusion can be caused by the idea that it is important to 'show commitment to the specialty'. But what does 'showing commitment' really mean? It is unlikely that commitment means applying for just one specialty—otherwise the system would discourage multiple applications. More likely, what is needed is that you demonstrate, within each application, how your experience to date equips you to train in that particular specialty.

> ## Box 6.5 **A doctor in no particular hurry**
>
> Cameron came into medicine as a mature student having done a first degree in molecular biology. In his first degree, Cameron had found himself intrigued by the medics' activities and responsibilities. This wasn't an obsession and Cameron had thoroughly enjoyed his own student life. But upon qualifying, Cameron began to look for ways to apply his subject matter to people's lives. He hadn't particularly enjoyed the lab work he'd done in his first degree. He also worried that if he went down a scientific or industry route, the subject matter might feel too narrow or too commercial.
>
> Cameron was successful in applying for a four-year medical course. You would think that after F2 Cameron might now have been eager to apply for training. However, he took the scenic route: an F3 year and as no decision seemed to make itself, a further year, F4, in the emergency department and on the wards of a large hospital.
>
> For a while Cameron shortlisted eight specialties. Over quite a long period, he whittled down the shortlist, applying for just three: psychiatry, general practice, and IMT. For each, Cameron was sure that further options could later open up—including occupational medicine, pharmaceutical medicine, and clinical neurophysiology.

One 'run-through' or two 'uncoupled' trainings?

Training in some specialties can be achieved via different training pathways: a single 'run-through' (with a single selection process in one geographic area) or alternatively two separate stages: so-called 'uncoupled' core and specialty trainings.

At the time of writing, for the acute specialties, a rotation of anaesthetics, intensive care medicine, emergency medicine and acute medicine is offered as a combined core training: the Acute Care Common Stem (ACCS). ACCS takes a year longer than core training in one or other specialty but allows for the development of a broader set of skills so, it is argued, doctors may become strong applicants to compete for the next leg of the training.

In psychiatry, run-through pilots allow trainees to sub-specialize from the outset in Child and Adolescent Psychiatry or Learning Disability Psychiatry. Alternatively, applicants can keep their options open by following a core psychiatry training, later following a sub-specialty within their specialty training.

Alternatives of this kind can create tricky choices. It can be worth envisioning how the specialty's membership exams will fit into the stages of training. If you feel bamboozled by the choice, it won't surprise you that we suggest re-visiting your own personal job criteria—the criteria in which you set out what was most important for you. You may, of course, have changed your view as to what's important so can revise your criteria.

Box 6.6 **Person specifications**

Most doctors are well aware that the centralized application system *Oriel* has links to the detailed person specifications for the specialty training programmes. These specify:

Eligibility criteria

These are the criteria you need to fulfil to be considered. They can be basic: having a primary medical degree; language skills; being registered or due to be registered with the regulatory body (the GMC). There can be a requirement not to have already trained in the specialty, not to be re-entering the specialty and not to have more than a defined number of years' experience in the specialty. If your own position is quite complex, we suggest making contact with a person involved in the selection process for that particular specialty.

Selection criteria

Divided into essential and desirable criteria, the selection criteria are those used to rank applicants. For each criterion, there is a minimum standard. Applicants ranked highest are first offered their choice of posts. Selection criteria include clinical skills, teaching, audit, quality improvement projects or research, personal qualities, and commitment to specialty. How the judgement is made is usually specified—whether through the application form, the MSRA exam or by interviewing applicants (often at an assessment centre). In practice interviews are a kind of exam.

If the conundrum remains stubborn, you could dip back into Chapter 5 to try an options appraisal, listen to your misgivings, or reconsider Fredkin's paradox.

It's now time to consider some of the specific rules of the game. We start in Box 6.6 with the recruiters' own criteria that make up the Person Specification.

The application itself

The experience of preparing for the selection process will differ depending on how much time you have. With a long lead time, there may still be time to gain a particular experience to strengthen your application. If you are preparing weeks or days before the deadline, you will be searching through the experiences you already have for ways in which you fulfil the selection criteria. Either way, it's helpful to keep physical or electronic folders of documentary evidence.

Application forms usually cut off at the number of words or characters specified. Try to be specific and factual, avoiding subjective claims and repetition. The assessor will make up their own mind based on your evidence. Given the importance of probity in medical practice, it's not surprising that it also counts a great deal in the selection process. With this need in mind, give a clear account of any gaps in your work history.

Box 6.7 **Written applications**

Good Medical Practice forms the bedrock for all medical specialties at all levels. As each of the four domains or 'pillars' is so central, it makes sense to cover all of them in the information you give about yourself: (1) Knowledge, skills and performance (2) Safety & quality (3) Communication, partnership and teamwork and (4) Maintaining trust. As the specialties periodically change the information they ask for in applications, it's important to check the selection criteria.

Audit and Quality Improvement Projects

Hopefully you participated in a project so can give an account of it, its relevance, your own role, and how the learning was shared. If the audit cycle was, or soon will be completed, you might earn extra points but don't be disheartened if that was not possible. You may be able to gain points through evidence of reflection and learning.

Presentations

If you presented a topic to a national, international or a local audience, orally or with a poster, include this information, stating your own role.

Publications

If you were fortunate to have been involved in original research and achieved a publication, give an account of this, outlining your own role.

Teaching

If you collected written feedback on any teaching you carried out, upload this as evidence. If you attended any courses on teaching, upload the evidence with reflections where possible.

Training courses

Training courses required for the specialty will likely score higher than those deemed less relevant. Honours, distinctions, or prizes in your primary medical qualification, or through a college or society may be invited.

Commitment to specialty

There are many ways to demonstrate your interest in the specialty: an elective or student-selected module, a taster day or week, membership of a society, attendance at a course or conference—even sitting part of an exam. As already discussed, commitment does not need to extend only to one specialty.

> ### Management and leadership skills
>
> Many types of experience can demonstrate management or leadership skills. Organizing a rota may seem a thankless task, but if you have had this role, you'll know how important it was for the service. Consider the skills you developed. Various types of activity at work, university or in leisure can help you develop skills in speaking, writing, motivating others, problem-solving, and much more.

At the same time, it's important to show your best self rather than under-selling yourself. To guard against this, ask a trusted friend or relative to read your draft application. A second pair of eyes can help you correct spelling or formatting errors, making your application look more professional.

Most readers will already be familiar with the information in Box 6.7, offered here for the sake of completion.

Exams

The Multi-Specialty Recruitment Assessment (MSRA), a computer-based exam was introduced in 2013 and was used widely during the pandemic. The Clinical Problem-solving section assesses clinical knowledge while the Professional Dilemmas section assesses your professional judgement in situations that can be encountered. Different specialties use the MSRA exam differently. In 2022, the MSRA score was the only criterion for selecting doctors into General Practice and Core Psychiatry training. Some specialties including Obstetrics & Gynaecology and Clinical Radiology use MSRA scores to shortlist applicants. For obstetrics and gynaecology (O&G), the highest scorers receive offers on their MSRA score alone. Some specialties do not use MSRA at all. Over time, specialties change and refine their assessment methods.

It can feel disheartening that exams crop up so often in medicine. But the evidence from psychology is unequivocal: ability tests predict future work performance more reliably than do subjective assessment methods like the traditional interview.[13] Painful as the prospect of another exam may be, there is a rationale for its use.

Though exams seem to be a constant, doctors lives do change. You may be busier and have less access to a peer group of candidates than you did as a student. If you can study with a peer group, as well as sharing resources, doing so you may allow you to enhance each other's self-efficacy. So it's worth the extra effort of searching out other doctors with whom to study.

Interviews and selection centres

'Traditional' interviews are still frequently used for doctors who, having trained, are applying for consultant or GP posts. The kind of interview that is similar to an OSCE (Objective Structured Clinical Examination) are really exams in all but name. As we have argued, they are fairer and more accurate. Another advantage is that they can be prepared for. In a helpful 'how-to' article, Rohman[14] discusses how he succeeded in attaining a training place in Orthopaedics. The strategies suggested would work across specialties. They include researching the process, timetabling, recruiting support from seniors and peers, anticipating questions, practising skills (videorecorded if possible), and filling gaps.

In non-medical interviews, the STAR acronym is often used to structure responses to questions like, 'Tell me about a situation when you …'. The STAR acronym prompts the applicant to speak about the **S**ituation facing them, then discuss the **T**ask they tackled. They progress to deal with how they **A**cted and finish up with the **R**esult or **R**eflection. The **R** stage demonstrates that you reflect and learn from experience. A different structure for answering questions might work just as well—but applying *a structure* to your answers can help with managing anxiety or can hold overconfidence in check. There is the added bonus of giving the interviewer a structure for listening to what you are saying.

What if I have a disability?

Figure 6.1 is intended as a reminder that the Equality Act 2010 requires selection panels to make reasonable adjustments to enable those with disabilities to perform at their best.

For reasonable adjustments to be made, you first need to make your needs known. The application form should invite you to answer affirmatively about any disability you may have, and the adjustments you think you need. You may feel more confident to state your needs if your needs have been assessed. The process of assessment should increase your confidence to ask for reasonable adjustments not only for the selection process but also for the work role itself. In addition to occupational health services, valuable information and support can be provided by the British Medical Association (BMA) and Access to Work (see their website at the end of the chapter).

Here are some adjustments that might be considered reasonable, depending upon the situation:

- You may need additional time to read a case study or be provided with accessible reading materials
- If you are physically unable to carry out certain procedures, being assessed 'by proxy' entails giving verbal instructions to another person
- Equipment may need to be adapted
- The position of the patient or equipment may need adjusting

Over time, progress has been made allowing doctors with disabilities to make significant contributions to the medical workforce. We are now becoming familiar with adjustments that would have been unimaginable in the past.

Alternative ways to train: the portfolio route

What about those doctors who choose *not* to apply for a formal training programme right away or even at all? It is definitely possible to have a satisfying career in a

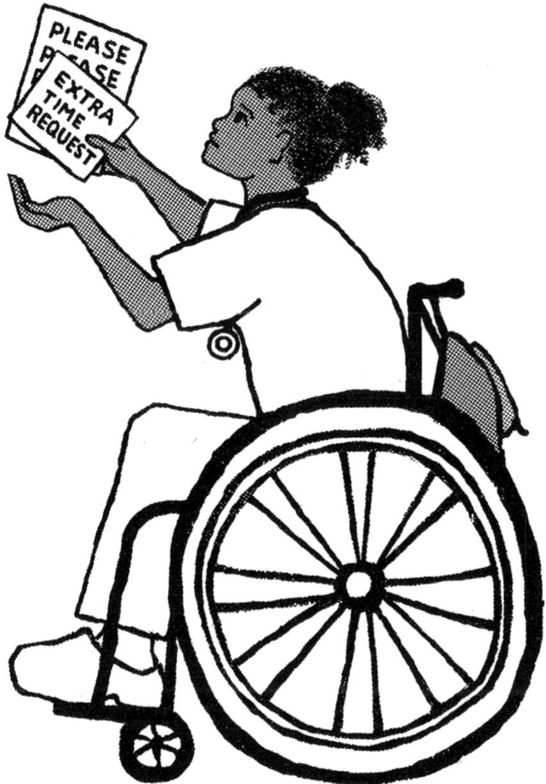

Figure 6.1 The Equality Act in practice.

non-training role. Moreover, for those doctors who go down this route, there is an alternative training pathway to becoming a consultant or GP: the portfolio route.

The UK has seen an expansion in the number of non-training posts.[11] Staff and Associate Specialist (SAS) and Locally Employed (LE) doctor roles have been replaced with Specialty Doctor roles with the expectation of doctors progressing to Specialist Doctor roles (not to be confused with consultant roles). The rise of the non-training roles is sometimes seen as a less expensive way of providing healthcare as these doctors' salaries are lower.[12] Nonetheless, non-training posts remain popular with doctors wanting to pause their training, and with doctors new to the UK. The duties are oriented towards the routine clinical work with less emphasis on balance, variety, or rotation. There may be a lesser commitment to the provision of out-of-hours on-call, such duties typically falling to those in training posts.

It is important to be aware that in the first of the General Medical Council (GMC)'s surveys of doctors SAS and LE posts, doctors in non-training roles were less likely than other doctors to feel well-supported and more likely to experience burn-out or to feel frustrated or bullied.[15] Just over a quarter of doctors in non-training posts had either applied or intended to apply to follow a 'Portfolio' route—the common term for the Certificate of Eligibility for Specialist Registration (CESR). CESR is a route by which a doctor can join the specialist register in recognition of skills evidenced through a portfolio. The equivalent Certificate of Eligibility for GP Registration (CEGPR) allows doctors with the requisite skills to join the GP register.

Our case study, Jacqui (Box 6.8) is an example of a doctor who followed the portfolio route.

Box 6.8 When life gets in the way of your art

Jacqui is a consultant haematologist working 8 PAs in Wales. Having completed a full-on Core Medical Training, Jacqui took the difficult decision *not* to continue training. Instead she applied for a 'middle grade' (non-training) post. At the time, Jacqui and her husband planned to adopt twins. It was thought the twins may have very significant additional needs. The plan was for each parent to care for their children two days each week with Jacqui's parents taking the children on the fifth day. It was important to Jacqui that her children's experience of growing up would be as good as her own. Jacqui doubted that a specialty training post would afford her the flexibility she wanted. She assumed a consultant role would be just as inflexible. She particularly wanted a break from on-call duties—at least for a few years.

Working as a middle grade doctor over many years allowed Jacqui to support her children in the way she wanted. And as she worked alongside the consultants, Jacqui became a skilled haematologist. She attended teaching with the haematology specialty trainees who became good friends. Later on, Jacqui had a reasonable continuous professional development (CPD) budget. Jacqui took on teaching responsibilities in a clinical area that was unpopular with colleagues. The specialism brought Jacqui into contact with staff from other parts of the hospital. Several colleagues commented that Jacqui was 'a consultant in all but name'. Quite often the haematology consultants asked Jacqui's opinion, not only in her specialist area but also in other areas.

All this led Jacqui to decide to follow a portfolio route. She felt she owed it to herself to be properly paid for her expertise. She also wanted to be a good role model for her children. It was easy to convince her colleagues who could see that when Jacqui was a consultant she would take a share in the on-call duties and in the supervision of the trainees.

The CESR process was a surprisingly rewarding process though it was not easy. Accumulating the necessary competencies and completing the paperwork took almost 3 years. But Jacqui found it less bureaucratic than adopting children! Soon after Jacqui was awarded her CESR, the NHS trust underwent a period of change. Two seniors retired, and Jacqui was the obvious person to lead the team. The trust offered a consultant role at a generous point on the pay scale, recognizing Jacqui's accumulated experience.

Taking a non-training path can be a very positive choice. The GMC survey of doctors in non-training roles[13] showed that most doctors who followed the CESR/CEGPR route felt supported in their career development by their organization. Receiving support and guidance really does seem to be crucially important.

Possible barriers to success in applications

Barrier No. 1: The differential attainment gap

We have known for some time that students who identify as Black and minority ethnic (BME) are disadvantaged in terms of educational attainment. This pattern occurs across all academic disciplines—including medicine. In a meta-analysis taking in nearly 24,000 candidates across 24 studies,[16] a significant difference of medium effect size, was shown between the attainments of white and non-white candidates. The findings apply irrespective of the exam type, level, and marking method. The problem of differential attainment also applies to specialty recruitment, and to doctors' progress (or lack of progress) in the Annual Review of Competency Progression (ARCP) process.[17]

Leading researcher in the field, Professor Kath Woolf, highlighted that the differentials are not caused by anything lacking in the BME students and trainees themselves. Her research suggests it is the day-to-day social interactions between students, teachers, and peers that critically affects their attainment. These social interactions are patterned by ethnicity.[18] Similarly, the late Dame Clare Marx, in her role as GMC Chair, highlighted the GMC finding that BME doctors' experience of medicine differs to that of their white colleagues, BME doctors receiving less support and feeling less able to raise concerns.[19]

The impetus for change must come from the organizations themselves so it is heartening that the GMC is now taking a lead to address the issue of differential attainment. But individuals can improve their chances by seeking the support of peers and seniors who believe in them and can provide the feedback and encouragement they deserve.

Barrier No. 2: Procrastination

Indecision can occur at any stage of career planning. When indecision sets in, it's tempting not to apply at all. If you notice this happening, it's worth re-visiting your own personal work criteria or repeating some of the exercises. Doing so may feel like time-wasting but ultimately you may end up saving time.

Remaining stuck or going round in circles may suggest the need for some career support. Local education training boards (LETBs) in England and deaneries in the rest of the UK provide career support, posting information about their services on their websites. Doctors can self-refer or be referred by their educational supervisor. Either way, career support should be available for trainees.

Barrier No. 3: Time pressure

Time pressure or being 'time-poor' (as most doctors are) can become a potent barrier to progressing with plans. But most doctors *do* prepare effectively for exams, and applying for training posts has a lot in common with exams. If you notice you're feeling time-poor, consider forming a planning group with peers to share strategies and hold each other to account. Some of the time management strategies discussed in Chapter 4 could be helpful in this scenario.

Summary

In this chapter we have considered the nuts and bolts of turning your career decision into reality. It may feel somewhat overwhelming as a lot can hinge on getting it right. For this reason we discussed general and career self-efficacy as well as some of the ways you may be able to boost your own career self-efficacy.

We discussed in detail some of the practical challenges because many doctors attending our seminars have asked for this. But the caveat is that things do change. So it's really important to check the way things are currently working in order to ensure that your understanding of what is required is up-to-date.

In considering the barriers to making a successful application, we dwelt particularly on the attainment gap. There is a tremendous obligation on the profession to improve inclusion and ultimately remove the attainment gap. Hopefully the wheels are already in motion. Meanwhile we hope that our discussion can embolden individuals to identify role models and construct a support team around themselves to good effect. Doing so may even expedite a process of bottom-up culture-change.

With notable exceptions, people find applications *hard*. The process of writing this chapter brought back our own memories of being under the microscope, and the inevitable imposter feelings that ensue. Our sense is there's little option but to master the rules and throw yourself into playing the game.

References

1. **Sharot, T.** (2011). The optimism bias. *Curr Biol.* **21**(23):R941–R945. DOI: 10.1016/j.cub.2011.10.030

2. **Kennedy, C.** (2015). Specialty training applications for entry in 2016: competition ratios and the application process. *BMJ.* **351**:h6005. https://doi.org/10.1136/bmj.h6005

3. **Burkeman, O.** (2021). *Four thousand weeks: time management for mortals.* Penguin, Random House.

4. **Bandura, A.** (1978). Self-efficacy: toward a unifying theory of behavioral change. *Adv Behav Res Ther.* **I**(4):139–161. https://doi.org/10.1016/0146-6402(78)90002-4

5. **Lent, R.W., & Hackett, G.** (1987). Career self-efficacy: Empirical status and future directions. *J Vocat Behav.* **30**(3):347–382. https://doi.org/10.1016/0001-8791(87)90010-8

6. **Chatterjee, D., Jacob, G.A., . . . & Chaudhary, S.** (2023). Career self-efficacy disparities in under-represented biomedical scientist trainees. *Plos One.* **18**(3):e0280608. https://doi.org/10.1371/journal.pone.0280608

7. **Moynihan, L.M., Roehling, M.V., . . . & Boswell, W.R.** (2003). A longitudinal study of the relationships among job search self-efficacy, job interviews, and employment outcomes. *J Bus Psychol.* **18**:207–233. https://doi.org/10.1023/A:1027349115277

8. **Saks, A.M.** (2006). Multiple predictors and criteria of job search success. *J Vocat Behav.* **68**(3):400–415. https://doi.org/10.1016/j.jvb.2005.10.001

9. **Petruzziello, G., Mariani, M.G., . . . & Guglielmi, D.** (2021). Self-efficacy and job search success for new graduates. *Pers Rev.* **50**(1):225–243. https://doi.org/10.1108/PR-01-2019-0009

10. **Carr, A., Marvell, J., & Collins, J.** (2013). Applying to specialty training: considering the competition. *BMJ*, **347**. DOI: https://doi.org/10.1136/bmj.f6568

11. **General Medical Council.** (2020, November). *The state of medical education and practice in the UK.* https://www.gmc-uk.org/-/media/documents/somep-2020_pdf-84684244.pdf

12. **Oxtoby, K.** (2010). The new lost tribe. *BMJ*, **341**. https://doi.org/10.1136/bmj.c5326

13. **Schmidt, F.L., & Hunter, J.E.** (1998). The validity and utility of selection methods in personnel psychology: Practical and theoretical implications of 85 years of research findings. *Psychological Bulletin*, **124**(2), 262. https://doi.org/10.1037/0033-2909.124.2.262

14. **Rohman, L.** (2015). My route to the golden ticket: securing a national training number in trauma and orthopaedics. *BMJ*, **351**, h3897. https://doi.org/10.1136/bmj.h3897

15. **General Medical Council.** (2020, January). *Specialty, associate specialist and locally employed doctors workplace experiences survey: Initial findings report.* https://www.gmc-uk.org/-/media/documents/sas-and-le-doctors-survey-initial-findings-report-060120_pdf-81152021.pdf

16. **Woolf, K., Potts, H.W., & McManus, I. C.** (2011). Ethnicity and academic performance in UK trained doctors and medical students: systematic review and meta-analysis. *BMJ.* **342**. https://doi.org/10.1136/bmj.d901

17. **General Medical Council** (2016). *How do doctors progress through key milestones during training?* https://www.gmc-uk.org/-/media/documents/How_do_doctors_progress_through_key_milestones_in_training.pdf_67018769.pdf

18. **Woolf, K.** (2020). Differential attainment in medical education and training. *BMJ.* **368**. https://doi.org/10.1136/bmj.m339

19. **General Medical Council** (2020). *Dame Clare Marx's message to the profession.* https://www.gmc-uk.org/news/news-archive/dame-clare-marxs-message-to-the-profession

Further reading

Dweck, C. (2017). *Mindset: changing the way you think to fulfil your potential.* Ballantine Books.

Further information

Academy of Medical Royal Colleges https://www.aomrc.org.uk/

Access to Work https://www.gov.uk/access-to-work

British Association of Sport and Exercise Medicine https://basem.co.uk/

Joint Committee on Surgical Training https://www.jcst.org/introduction-to-training/

Medical Training Recruitment https://medical.hee.nhs.uk/medical-training-recruitment/medical-specialty-training/person-specifications

NHS Health Careers https://www.healthcareers.nhs.uk/explore-roles/explore-roles

Oriel https://www.oriel.nhs.uk/Web/

Royal College of Psychiatrists https://www.rcpsych.ac.uk/become-a-psychiatrist

SAS Doctor Development https://www.aomrc.org.uk/wp-content/uploads/2020/10/SAS_doctor_development_guide_1020.pdf

Specialty Training Competition Ratios https://www.specialty-applications.co.uk/competition-ratios/

The Society for Acute Medicine https://www.acutemedicine.org.uk/

Chapter 7

Succeeding as an international medical graduate

We now want to consider the needs of international medical graduates (IMGs)—doctors who qualified in a country other than that in which they intend to practice. In considering the needs of IMGs we include the need to welcome IMGs into the domestic health economy. Our five-stage approach to career planning applies as much to IMGs as to everyone else. You'll recall these stages are more iterative than linear. For reasons we will discuss, the need for iteration is more important for those who are changing country. The exploration stage is an altogether bigger project than it is for local graduates. In this chapter we describe some of the 'anatomy' of UK healthcare—with the caveat that what we describe will need supplementing with more up-to-date information. We end by discussing the barriers faced by IMGs in considerable detail.

Why are IMGs important?

The day-to-day working of the NHS depends on doctors and nurses who initially trained outside the UK. According to the General Medical Council (GMC) workforce survey[1] the number of doctors from outside the European Economic area working in the UK rose by 267% between 2016 and 2021. Domestically, the increase in the number of UK medical student places (135% over five years) is insufficient to take care of the needs of the UK's ageing population.[2] Doctors often choose to work in the UK to develop their skills and their careers. In Chapter 11 we show that many UK doctors choose to work abroad for the same reason. The need to utilize the skills of doctors trained elsewhere is not unique to the UK. Other Western countries also depend upon doctors from around the world. But it means that the 'donor' countries then experience shortages of health professionals.[3]

In theory, the reciprocal sets of needs of the health economy and doctors should make career-planning relatively straightforward. But of course nothing is ever simple!

The stages of career decision-making revisited

Here, we revisit the five stages introduced in Chapter 1, and the exercises within the first self-knowledge stage (set out in Chapter 2). While not detailing the exercises here, we do discuss how they can be adapted to meet different needs. It is, however, worth reiterating that the self-knowledge stage is analogous to the history-taking stage of clinical care. Its aim is to make explicit your implicit self-knowledge.

Stage 1: Self-knowledge

The values exercise

In the values exercise we invite you to rank-order a set of work values that are relevant to medical careers. You're likely to rank the values differently in different contexts. In one country, for example, working in the community might entail delivering healthcare to a remote, rural community. In another, a community setting could be quite different. Another consideration is your own changing needs. You might thrive working autonomously in the country in which you graduated. But as you consider forging the whole or part of a career in an entirely new health setting, your priorities may change. The case study in Box 7.1 and Table 7.1 illustrates this point.

Our values often change with time and place. The values exercise is quick and easy to do, so can be repeated.

The experience log

The experience log is simply a log of your experiences, noted soon after episodes occur. It's an opportunity to reflect on what experiences were like and what your experience might mean for your future. Changing priorities show themselves in this exercise too. While you may have felt fulfilled working autonomously in your home country, a clinical attachment in a new country can lead you to experience confusion or frustration. As a newcomer in a country, carrying out the experience log may tell you more about

---

Box 7.1 Repeating the values exercise

As an internship doctor in Bangladesh, Hassan wanted to train as thoroughly as possible. As a student, he was involved in a research project mapping the needs of the rural elderly population. Hassan could see that rural populations needed far better information about the common conditions like diabetes and stroke—what to look out for and when to seek medical assistance. A distal aim was to be trained to be able to set up services with integrated health education—for the population and the professionals.

In spite of the intensity of his internship year, Hassan found time to explore career options. He was accepted onto a distance-learning MSc course that could run alongside a postgraduate training. He looked to the UK and knew the process would be competitive and lengthy.

Hassan twice carried out the values exercise (Table 7.1). At each stage 'Contact with patients' and 'Helping people' were top-ranking values. However, as Hassan learnt about the NHS and training in the UK, and recalling the more overwhelming side of being an intern, Hassan now saw 'Supervision', 'Predictability', and 'Hospital setting' as important. Thinking about the care he wanted one day to deliver, 'Variety' also became important. But in an unfamiliar setting, he needed to consider how work and studying would work together.

Table 7.1 Changes in Hassan's values exercise ratings

Ranking	Thinking about practising in home country	Thinking about practising in new country
1st most important	Contact with patients	Contact with patients
2nd most important	Helping people	Helping people
3rd most important	Variety	Supervision
4th most important	Being expert	Being expert
5th most important	Learning	Learning
6th most important	Teaching	Predictability
7th most important	Supervision	Hospital setting
8th most important	Work with others	Teaching

your wellbeing and support needs. For *career planning*, the experience log is more valuable once you feel more settled.

The achievements exercise

The achievements exercise encourages you to think about your achievements. For most of us it's important to build on our strengths and interests. This may seem too obvious to need stating but we have sometimes worked with doctors who built their careers on topics that made them highly anxious. Of course there can be real value in facing our fears but this does not necessarily mean that we should opt for a career option that we find highly stressful.

One reason it's important to find a natural fit with your own natural skills is that IMGs often have to compete with doctors who trained in their home country. UK graduates will have developed an intuitive awareness of the workings of the NHS and training. IMGs must first learn how things work in their home country, then the workings of the system in their new country. The differential attainment gap (discussed in the 'Possible barriers to progressing as an IMG' section at the end of this chapter and Chapter 6) is such that the playing field is not a level one. So it makes sense to play to your strengths rather than playing with one hand tied behind your back.

But it can be difficult to judge your own strengths and abilities. In Chapter 8 we discuss why it's common to either over-rate or under-rate your own abilities. Because accurate self-appraisal is so hard, you might consider supplementing your own self-appraisal with feedback from a supportive senior who knows your work. Peers can also provide useful feedback or you can reflect on feedback you already have.

- What do your peers and seniors consider your strengths to be? In what areas do they see you struggle?

- What achievements have you made that aroused admiration, pride, or even others' envy?

- What personal aptitudes or qualities do your peers or seniors recognize in you?

- What feedback have you received (or what feedback could you ask for) that may point to your strengths and abilities?

Career lifeline, writing exercise, and drawing exercises

The career lifeline, writing, and drawing exercises aid reflection. As you turn your mind to each exercise, consider which of your past experiences may be relevant to the plans you are now formulating. Perhaps you previously studied or worked some distance from your family. If so, what was that experience like? How did you manage the transitions? What support did you need?

Stage 2: Exploration

We normally suggest first explicating one's 'inner' self-knowledge, then exploring the 'out there' opportunities. For IMGs the process is more iterative and the exploration is wider as it includes such issues as visas, medical registration, and language tests.

Consider if your exploration so far has been based on information from formal or informal sources. By informal, we mean information from peers, peer websites, and commercial companies. By formal we mean the information on 'official' websites—written by those responsible for training and recruitment. These should be more reliable sources of information about the 'rules of the game'. Though reliable, the formal sources can be thin on the practical ideas that peers can offer. So both sources are important.

The information in this chapter—and in this book—comes with a health warning: it will become outdated, so it's also vital to search out up-to-date information.

Shortlisting options

You'll recall that the shortlisting stage is equivalent to the differential diagnosis stage of clinical care. You are listing the options you plan to look into. Consider:

- whether you plan to return to your home country. If so, what skills, qualifications, and experience do you want or need to take with you?

- what specialties might you be well-suited to and find rewarding?

- Do you hope to train to be a general practitioner (GP), a consultant, or to apply for a non-training post? Specialty training is not for everybody at every moment. Prior to training, many doctors first familiarize themselves with the country, culture, and healthcare system in a non-training post. Doing so positions them to apply for a training programme or to follow the portfolio (CESR) route. If you plan to apply to a training programme, it may be important to avoid gaining so much experience that you become ineligible to train. Some specialties set an upper limit for how much specialty experience applicants can have prior to training.

Stage 3: Investigation

The investigation stage involves carrying out a structured enquiry into each of your shortlisted options. By asking searching questions, you go beyond the information given on the websites. It's tempting to adopt an incognito approach, relying exclusively on the online information. For one thing, it may be hard to find contact details for key people and harder to summon up the courage to approach them. But against this, consider that in some hospitals it *is* possible to be introduced to an approachable consultant or doctor in the latter stages of their training. As an IMG you will have more questions than local graduates. For everybody, IMG and UK-graduate alike, it's wise to prepare a list of questions in advance rather than leaving the conversation to chance.

Stage 4: Career plan

Making your career plan is the career-planning equivalent of making a diagnosis. When dealing with diagnostic issues in clinical practice, you generally factor in the prevalence of the conditions you're considering. In career planning, this translates to factoring in in the number of available training posts and the competition ratios. These will determine how many specialties you might want to apply to.

Stage 5: Implementation

Being equivalent to the 'management' in clinical care, the implementation stage involves preparing for, and applying for posts. If you're unsuccessful the first time round, you may need to apply again. It's helpful to ask for feedback which you can then discuss with trusted seniors. Support or mentoring (sometimes available within the NHS) is very valuable. Mentoring may also be available through one of the professional associations for international doctors, listed at the end of the chapter.

Anatomy of UK medical careers

Having outlined the career-planning stages, we now return to the exploration stage to discuss some of the issues that need exploring.

UK careers tend to proceed along predetermined pathways shown in Figure 7.1. Most training takes place in NHS settings, so IMGs are well-advised to look to NHS posts to gain their initial experience upon entering the UK. There is often an early need to learn how clinical services are organized, as well as the broader culture of healthcare services.

From this vantage point, the questions posed in Chapter 3 can now be tackled. What conditions and treatments are particular to the specialty? Are the specialty's skills those you would like to acquire? How compatible are they with your own interests and aptitudes? How specialized or varied is the work in that particular specialty? Is the work done in a setting that fits with your own preferences? How competitive is it to get a training place in that specialty?

There will also be areas for exploration that concern life outside work. Where would you prefer to live and work? What is the demographic make-up of the community in that geographic area? Could the area meet your religious or spiritual needs? If you have a family, what are the local schools like? It's easy to neglect sport, leisure, and transport.

Language tests

The GMC accepts two equivalent language tests: International English Language Testing System (IELTS) and Occupational English Test (OET). Both cover reading,

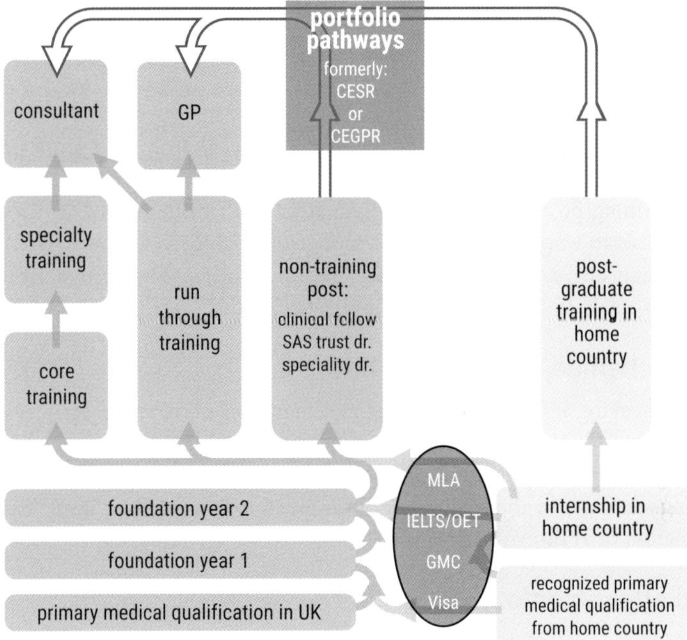

Figure 7.1 UK career pathways.

writing, speaking, and listening. IELTS tests language skills to an academic standard. Universities typically require students to score 5.5 to 6, while doctors must usually score an average of 7.5, with a scores of 7 or more for each domain. The OET aims to assess health professionals' language and communication skills so set clinically relevant topics. Doctors must score B in each domain. A study of 50 refugee doctors familiar with both testing systems showed a preference for the OET.[4] The doctors found the language tested by OET to be more relevant which enhanced both their motivation and their chance of passing.

The PLAB

The Professional and Linguistic Assessment Board (PLAB) has two stages. PLAB 1, an applied knowledge test, can be sat in countries outside the UK. PLAB 2, an objective structured clinical exam (OSCE) is conducted at UK clinical assessment centres. The skills tested are those expected of doctors who have completed the first year of the UK foundation programme.

Registration

In the UK, the GMC is the organization that determines whether a primary medical qualification is recognized. Doctors seeking work as a foundation doctor F1 post apply for 'provisional registration' while those who have completed internships elsewhere, including those applying for 'standalone F2 posts' apply for 'full registration'.

Registration occurs when a language test and the PLAB 2 have been passed. The GMC also grants a licence to practice.

Visas

The UK visa requirements changed following the UK's exit from the European Union. At the time of writing, medicine was seen as a shortage occupation, allowing IMGs to apply for training posts alongside UK graduates. The Health and Care Worker Visa enables doctors to work in the UK, performing 'an eligible job with the NHS or NHS supplier'. Practically, a confirmed job offer is needed, the employer providing a certificate of sponsorship to support the visa application.

Special schemes

It's worth checking if there are any special schemes to make the process easier. For doctors planning to return to a lower income country, the Medical Training Initiative (MTI) offers two-year programmes of specialist training. But it is important to be aware that schemes like the MTI do not train doctors to consultant level (Certificate of Completion of Training, CCT).

Clinical attachments

A clinical attachment is an observational post with no clinical responsibilities. Such positions are normally unpaid, or may charge a fee for the experience. Attachments allow IMGs to build networks, learn about the NHS, gain experience in clinical audit, find out about a particular specialty and make yourself known. It is sometimes possible to arrange for an attachment to coincide with a visit for the PLAB 2.

The foundation programme

UK medical graduates follow a two-year programme of supervised experience, the foundation programme which replaced the one-year internship that many countries still have. Foundation doctors typically rotate through three posts each year. The foundation years allow doctors to experience several specialties. Some foundation programmes include general practice, psychiatry, or surgery; some include academic research.

In theory IMGs can apply for the whole foundation programme or, following their internship at home, they could apply to a 'standalone F2 post' (though the availability of such posts does vary). To be eligible for a standalone F2 post, doctors need to achieve higher language test grades—7.5 in each IELT domain or 400 for each OET domain.

Upon completing the second Foundation Year (FY2) doctors are awarded a Foundation Programme Completion Certificate (FPCC). The equivalent skills can be demonstrated through the Certificate for Readiness to Enter Specialty Training (CREST) form, in which each skill observed is signed off by the supervising consultant. This can be a consultant supervisor in many home countries or for those in UK non-training posts, the UK consultant supervisor. As the rules for completion of the CREST form are exacting, it is important to check them with an official website such as that of Health Education England, listed at the end of the chapter.

Non-training posts

The UK has seen a steady growth in the number of its medical posts—and particularly the number of non-training posts.[1] Non-training posts are known by many different names: staff and associate specialist (SAS), specialty doctor, specialist, associate specialist, trust grade doctor, or locally employed doctor. Such posts are oriented to service delivery. The doctors in the posts are not part of an incremental training programme that leads to qualifying as a consultant. Clinical fellowships are non-training posts which are typically well-supervised. They attract doctors who, having completed their F2 year, want to top-up their experience and strengthen their training post applications.

Surprisingly, non-training medical posts don't yet exist in general practice. It is possible that the GMC will in the future support the development of such posts (alongside increases in the non-medical workforce).[5]

Training posts

The most common way to progress to becoming a consultant is to apply to a training programme. The competition is considerable. It's helpful to check the competition ratios for the preceding years—that is, the number of applicants per training post. As it is so important to demonstrate that you have the skills in each area of the GMC's guiding principles *Good Medical Practice*,[6] it is worth studying this document. Many of these skills can be refined while working in a non-training post.

Training programmes are categorized either as either 'run-through' or 'uncoupled'. Run-through training means the training is integrated into a single programme. Typically, doctors are appointed to the first year of the training: 'ST1'. With 'uncoupled training', appointments are first made to the 'CT1' stage of Core Training. Doctors later apply to enter specialty training, typically being appointed to 'ST 3' or 'ST4'. Progress is monitored through an Annual Review of Competence Progression (ARCP), the end goal being the CCT.

Consultant posts

Doctors awarded a CCT are listed in the GMC's specialist register or GP register and are eligible to apply for consultant or GP posts. Consultants deliver specialist healthcare alongside the doctors in training and doctors in non-training posts who they supervise. Consultants usually lead multidisciplinary teams of health professionals including nurses or midwives. But consultants don't supervise or line-manage the other health professionals; this is the responsibility of senior practitioners within each profession.

Though most IMGs enter the UK medical workforce at an early stage in their careers, it is also possible to enter the UK healthcare system at consultant or GP level. To do so, senior doctors must demonstrate the equivalence of their training, applying to the GMC to follow the portfolio (CESR or CEGPR) route.

General Practice

General Practice is a specialty in its own right in the UK. General Practitioners (GPs) treat common and long-term conditions and refer patients to hospitals or specialist teams when needed. The three-year training is the shortest specialty training. As well as being registered on the GMC GP register, GPs also need to register locally on the GP Performers' List.[7]

Recent years have seen shortages of GPs despite various initiatives to boost GP numbers.[8] Doctors who have trained and worked as GPs in their own country can apply to the Royal College of GPs for a Certificate of Eligibility for GP Registration (CEGPR).

The portfolio route

The CESR and CEGPR routes, discussed earlier, allow doctors to demonstrate the equivalence of their prior training. The CESR has also come to be used domestically as a more flexible alternative to regular training programmes. Doctors in substantive (permanent) non-training posts can apply to the GMC to follow the route, developing a portfolio of evidence of the required competencies. The portfolio is then assessed by the relevant Royal College. When the process goes well, a Certificate of Equivalence for Specialist Registration (CESR) is awarded. It is quite a lengthy process requiring great organization and commitment from both the individual and the employer. Increasingly NHS organizations are willing to consider—or plan for—a doctor following the CESR route.

The GP equivalent, the CEGPR is a way for those who trained in other countries to demonstrate the equivalence of their training.

The case study in Box 7.2 is based upon an article in the *Quarterly Journal of Medicine*.[9] Keen to encourage doctors with prior experience to follow the CESR route, Dr Mohammad Allaboudy has kindly given us permission to share his experience.

Mohammad's scenario can be seen as 'win-win' given the clear benefits for his NHS organization. A survey, published in 2017 found 77% of NHS employers struggling to recruit to non-training posts.[10] But NHS organizations which support doctors through the portfolio route are better able to recruit and retain their doctors.

The foregoing discussion is intended as an introduction to some of the posts likely to be encountered in the UK. The need to 'learn the anatomy' makes the exploration phase an altogether bigger project than it is for local graduates.

There is one particular group of international graduates for whom the project is more challenging still.

Refugee doctors

Refugee doctors are a group of IMGs whose situation has been affected by the need to flee a war zone or from the risk of persecution. Such an event can occur at any career stage. It follows that refugee doctors often have serious worries about family members and may experience mental health difficulties[11] or struggle with their sense of who they are.[12,13] Re-entering a professional role even at a level lower can mark the beginning of a recovery process. For many, it is hard to contemplate taking a job unrelated to medicine.

Box 7.2 **Getting prior experience and expertise recognized**

After training in Egypt in geriatric medicine, Mohammad could see that the structure of his training was quite different from UK training. Preparing to apply for a non-training post in the UK Midlands, Mohammad studied the websites. He knew he could, in theory, follow the CESR route to have his skills recognized. But he also knew he would need new skills to fit the new context. At interview, Mohammad spoke with clarity and enthusiasm about his previous work and the personal development plan he hoped to put in place. Mohammad's motivation was infectious: the interview panel wanted to support him. The NHS Trust identified a consultant mentor to help Mohammad navigate the CESR route. Mohammad gained experience in community geriatrics and in many specialist areas: old age psychiatry, ortho-geriatrics, movement disorders, continence, and much more. Mohmmad followed his Royal College evaluator's advice to use the electronic portfolio designed for trainees and he also used a project management tool to keep track of the gaps—and fill them.

The process was practically feasible but required considerable planning and flexibility on the part of the managers and Mohammad's colleagues. Within several months of submitting his initial portfolio, Mohammad had made the revisions necessary for the portfolio to be accepted. With Mohammad now named on the specialist register, the situation was win-win—for Mohammad and his NHS trust. The trust had an additional highly esteemed member of the consultant body. Mohammad was able to become a Fellow of the Royal College of Physicians. He now leads his department in several areas including its CESR training.

Data from Allaboudy, M., Ali, A., & Masud, T. (2018). Gaining a certificate of eligibility for specialist registration (CESR) in the UK. *QJM: An International Journal of Medicine*, 111 (suppl. 1), hcy200-068. https://doi.org/10.1093/qjmed/hcy200.068

Before taking the first step back towards medical practice, refugee doctors must first be granted asylum status. Unfortunately, the slowness of the UK asylum system can create significant gaps in doctors' work histories. To add to the complexity, not all primary medical qualifications and postgraduate trainings are recognized. Because the process is complex, refugees need local professional help from specialist organizations. We list a number at the end of the chapter. Those who apply for UK jobs without support seem to struggle more.[14] Support can allow the refugee doctor to:

- learn English to the required level
- engage in a personalized assessment of career needs
- receive support for CV-writing
- receive support or advocacy to enable them to meet the requirements of the professional organizations
- be signposted to organizations providing financial support for exams
- find a peer group to provide advice and support

- access work experience—which can be observational, hands-on (or both), paid or unpaid

You might wonder if such benefits are possible in reality. The Building Bridges Programme (Box 7.3) followed-up the doctors who had used their service.

The doctors' roles may often have been at a level lower than those their previous roles. But it's encouraging that the doctors were able to get a foothold. Without one, gaps might have opened up in the doctors' work histories that would be hard if not impossible to resolve.

With appropriate practical support, refugee doctors *can and do* find meaningful employment as doctors—though the route can be tortuous. This was the experience of Layla who we discuss in Box 7.4.

Given the shortage of doctors in the UK, it makes sense for practical support to be provided to refugee doctors and for it to be taken up by the doctors who make up this group. Doing so benefits everybody.

Possible barriers to progressing as an IMG

But there are many potential obstacles that face refugee doctors and IMGs more generally. Here we discuss two particular barriers that IMGs share with other doctors—those who identify as Black and minority ethnic (BAME or BME). They are the differential attainment gap and the differential referral gap. In discussing these issues, our intention is not to be alarmist but to raise doctors' awareness, increasing their chance of success and of being professionally safe.

> ### Box 7.3 **The Building Bridges Programme**
>
> NHS funded, the Building Bridges Programme also has links with the Refugee Council and the Refugee Assessment and Guidance Unit, and is hosted by London Metropolitan University. The Building Bridges Programme supports refugee health professionals in London. There are similar programmes in other areas in the UK.
>
> Eighty-five doctors working with the Clinical Apprenticeship Scheme (CAPS) from 2009 to 2020 were followed-up.[14] The scheme supported the doctors to work in supernumerary positions at F2 doctor level (their roles were additional to those of doctors normally employed). Forty-five (94%) of the doctors returning questionnaires now worked in the NHS:
>
> 21 (47% of the NHS employees) were employed as trust grade doctors
>
> 7 (17%) were GP trainees
>
> 6 (13%) were specialty trainees
>
> 5 (11%) worked in another capacity
>
> These doctors particularly valued the communication skills training they had received, as well as the emotional support provided, the local culture being so very different to that they had been used to.
>
> Data from Shah, R. et al., (2021). An evaluation of the CAPS refugee doctor scheme in London–a survey of outcomes. *Education for Primary Care*, 32(2), 100-103. DOI:10.108 0/14739879.2020.1857662

> ## Box 7.4 **A refugee doctor's experience**
>
> Layla works as an ST1 in General Practice. It is not many years since she was in her third year of medical school in Yemen and the civil war in Yemen developed, making it unsafe to remain. Layla's family reached Southeast Asia. Layla's best chance of completing her medical studies was in Jordan, thousands of miles from her family. Fortunately, Jordan was a welcoming country without any linguistic challenges and with a good cultural match. But Layla experienced a career challenge after qualifying and completing her internship. The number of medical posts was insufficient for refugee doctors like Layla to be permitted to apply.
>
> Layla found support through an International Medical Graduates' Facebook group. Proficient in English, Layla decided to sit the OET. This meant travelling to an exam centre in Egypt. Next stop was an exam centre in Pakistan for the PLAB 1. Upon arrival in the UK on a visitor visa for the PLAB 2, the COVID-19 pandemic set in. The exam was cancelled with no known future dates. Layla needed to decide whether to wait it out or return with little accomplished. One idea that proved impracticable was to apply for a healthcare assistant role, but no organization could sponsor Layla for a visa to work.
>
> Fearful of overstaying her visitor visa, Layla urgently needed advice. She could afford an hour of a solicitor's time. The rushed advice was to seek asylum: returning to Jordan, it was reasoned, might risk being returned to Yemen where doctors could be forced to care for the rebel militias. Alone in a foreign country, Layla's plan had been derailed. Layla fearfully wondered how her situation might look. After a long process involving a second legal opinion, political asylum was granted.
>
> During her year of waiting, Layal was not allowed to work. But Layla set herself challenging goals and reached out for help. A friend shared their Multi-Specialty Recruitment Assessment (MSRA) exam questions. The organizations REACH and Refugee Action provided career advice, CV help, signposting, and funded Layla's exams. Taking courage, Layla contacted numerous NHS consultants. As Layla started her clinical attachment at a nearby emergency department, her morale picked up. Finally she was doctoring again—gaining valuable hands-on experience in her adopted country.
>
> Now, training as a GP, Layla can look back and see that she made the very best use of her waiting period. She succeeded in passing two exams and undertook a clinical attachment. With support, she got her career back on track.

Barrier No. 1: The differential attainment gap

For medicine and most other subjects that can be studied, students' educational attainments are found to be lower if a student belongs to a minority ethnic group.[15] This is the differential attainment gap. Attainment gaps are demonstrated in postgraduate medical exams,[16,17] irrespective of whether the exam is marked by human or machine.

The Clinical Skills Assessment (CSA), now superseded by the Simulated Consultation Assessment (SCA) was the GP 'exit' exam. The CSA suffered from a differential between white and non-white doctors as well as a small differential between women and men, women tending to do better. But the greatest differential was between UK graduates and IMGs. The profession's awareness of the issue was heightened by a case being brought to judicial review by British Association of Physicians of Indian Origin (BAPIO). The judgement made in 2014 by the Honourable Mr Justice Mitting was that the practices had been lawful. There was a caveat: with reference to the Royal College of General Practitioners, Mr Justice Mitting said, 'If it does not act and its failure to act is the subject of a further challenge in the future, it may well be that it will be held to have breached its duty'.[18]

The CSA case is not unique. The Royal College of Psychiatrist's Clinical Assessment of Skills and Competencies (CASC) also has a significant attainment gap, a gradient in the pass rate having been demonstrated in a study of over 2,000 candidates' performance.[19] With 93% of white UK graduates passing first time, the corresponding figure for UK BME graduates was 79%. Fewer (57%) of European Economic Area (EEA) graduates passed first time. The group *least* likely to pass first time was doctors who had graduated outside the EEA—IMGs. This group's first-time pass rate was 29%.

Language may have been a factor, as the CASC scores and language scores correlated. But what else might contribute to the attainment gaps seen in postgraduate exams? A qualitative study examining the experience of doctors in training addresses this question.[20] Those UK graduates identifying as BME as well as IMGs experienced greater disadvantage, feeling less supported, and less believed by their seniors. Some BME UK graduates felt protected if they had graduated from a good UK medical school or if they spoke with middle class accents. In contrast, IMGs were more likely to feel their accent stood in their way. The UK way of doing things was different and the doctors needed to learn a great deal. Yet the doctors felt fearful of asking for help or taking extra courses—which could be perceived as a sign of weakness.

It is unavoidable that moving to a new healthcare system involves so much new learning. The country, its population and culture inevitably differ. Topics like consent, confidentiality, and end-of-life care will differ greatly across cultures.[21,22] The doctor–patient relationship, colleague relationships, and the culture of teaching and learning are also disparate.[23]

A GMC-commissioned study took a fresh and optimistic approach. Through focus groups comprising trainees from programmes that did not suffer from differential attainment gaps, *What supported your success in training?*[24] allows us to see beyond the difficulties often encountered. We can begin to learn what enables doctors identifying as BME to progress more comfortably. We summarize some of the themes that emerged in Box 7.5.

The findings resonate with the experience of Dr Chukwudi[25] who wrote a heartening personal account of his experience in a standalone F2 role (Box 7.6).

The foregoing discussion suggests several strategies that are worth trying:

- Attend inductions that are offered, talk to seniors and peers, whether they are IMGs or local graduates.
- Don't be afraid to ask questions.

◆ Take opportunities to teach in areas in which you feel confident—there will be topics about which you know more than your colleagues!

◆ Raise any difficulties with your supervisor. What if there is no supervisor? If supervision isn't provided, can supervision or mentoring be arranged? If an organization cannot provide support, might an alternative employer better meet your needs?

◆ At first you may need a little more time to accomplish tasks that would be easier for a home-grown doctor. Don't be afraid to raise this.

◆ In the spirit of Growth Mindset (discussed in Chapter 8), ask for feedback. As we discuss in Chapter 8, Growth Mindset is an orientation to learning: we learn more effectively when we can see our mistakes as learning opportunities.

Barrier No. 2: The differential referral gap

Regrettably the differentials are not limited to attainments. Differentials also occur in the likelihood of referral to the GMC, the regulatory organization.[26,27] Doctors whose primary qualification was awarded outside the UK are 2.5 times more likely to be referred to the GMC. UK graduates identifying as BME are twice as likely to be referred to the regulator.

Box 7.5 What supported your success in training?

◆ Diversity was 'visible' in the organizations that did not suffer from a Differential Attainment Gap. BME trainees felt represented when they saw senior colleagues as like themselves.

◆ Trainees felt confident, motivated, and inspired by seniors, who set high standards.

◆ Trainees felt they were treated as an individuals, supported to raise issues, and encouraged to develop.

◆ Trainees received feedback and were supported to be able to make sense of any negative experiences.

◆ Good learning experiences—such as exam preparation—occurred. When trainees did not pass exams, they were supported to understand what had gone wrong.

◆ Peers supported, advised, and helped each other make sense of working life and helped each other prepare for exams.

◆ Shifts and working patterns did not interfere with learning or with relationship-building.

◆ Trainees were supported with career planning and were supported to make strong applications.

Data from Roe, V et al. (2019). What supported your success in training?. A qualitative exploration of the factors associated with an absence of an ethnic attainment gap in post-graduate specialty training. GMC. https://www.gmc-uk.org/-/media/documents/gmc-da-final-report-success-factors-in-training-211119_pdf-80914221.pdf

> ### Box 7.6 **An IMG doctor's experience of being F2 doctor**
>
> 'In the initial four weeks, I did a lot of asking around, as I was new to the NHS system with so many things strange to me. I would encourage anyone starting out new in the system to ask as many questions [as you need to] and learn the most you can …
>
> 'A lot of things are going on at once: you are trying to adjust to a new country, you are learning an entirely new healthcare system, you are ticking off F2 standalone portfolio requirements and also trying to gather the necessary portfolio for GP or specialty applications, among other family or personal commitments. It can feel very overwhelming.
>
> Try to connect with F2 standalone trainees in other trusts, as this will help keep you grounded and provide a sense of community. Making an effort to connect with the F2s in your trust will also pay off as they will help signpost you to courses or resources available in your trust or deanery that you may not ordinarily learn about.'
>
> Reproduced from Chukwudi I, 'UKFPO F2 Standalone: A brief guide', *Annals of Medicine and Surgery*, 82. DOI: 10.1016/j.amsu.2022.104594. Copyright Wolters Kluwer

One particular case was widely publicized, informing our learning. Dr Arora graduated in India and worked in the UK as a locum doctor in primary care. In attempting to resolve an issue, Dr Arora argued that she had been offered the use of a laptop computer. In 2020, Dr Arora's employer referred Dr Arora to the GMC, concerned about the doctor's probity. A tribunal two years later found Dr Arora's fitness to practice to be 'impaired'. Dr Arora's licence to practice was removed—though only for a month. A storm erupted in the medical profession and in the media.[28] The GMC announced an independent review of their processes.[29] At an appeal heard at the High Court, the findings of the tribunal were overturned. There had been a mighty storm in a teacup. Some of the recommendations of the independent review that followed, 'Fair to Refer?' (2019)[30] are summarized in Box 7.7.

In a subsequent Independent Learning Review, the GMC was advised it should be encouraging concerned referrers to first involve their own 'Responsible Officer' (usually their medical director). Organizations could develop cultures of resolving issues locally before taking the step of referring a doctor to the medical regulator.

Had the recommendations of *Fair to Refer?* and the independent review been in place at the time, the story of Dr Arora's laptop might have developed very differently. With comprehensive support, an issue may not have arisen at all. Or if one did arise, it could have been resolved locally without any attribution of dishonesty being made.

The recommendations of *Fair to Refer?* are directed towards organizations. Systemic problems are the responsibility of systems, not individuals. But as an individual, you may wonder what you personally can do to reduce the risk of a complaint being made against you. As the potential consequences are so detrimental, it is worth wondering if you as an individual can prompt your organizations to provide the kind of support that is now recommended. It is, we acknowledge, difficult to accept help and even more difficult to *ask* for it. Yet it is vitally important to develop a good support network.

In Box 7.8 we suggest some steps that could help to resolve particularly difficult situations.

Box 7.7 **Recommendations of *Fair to Refer?***

1. Doctors new to the UK, to the NHS, or working in isolated posts should be comprehensively supported.

2. Senior leaders should engage regularly with all staff, listening to, and responding to staff concerns about fairness.

3. Seniors should introduce safeguards to resolve issues of bias and favouritism.

4. Systemic issues influencing performance should be addressed in such a way that if concerns around performance arise, the emphasis will be on learning rather than blame.

5. The GMC should monitor the degree to which referrals it receives are proportionate and should work to reduce the risk of disproportionate referrals.

Data from General Medical Council. (2019). Fair to Refer? Reducing disproportionality in fitness to practice concerns reported to the GMC. https://www.gmc-uk.org/-/media/documents/fair-to-refer-report_pdf-79011677.pdf

---

Box 7.8 **Suggested steps to resolving difficult issues**

1. If there is an issue you are worried about, decide who you could speak to. Could an informal meeting be arranged?

2. You might find it helpful to write a few notes as a memory aid. But if you do so, don't make your notes so formal or extensive that the meeting feels like an enquiry!

3. Talk about situations that worry you, about any effects the issue has on you—for example, if you find yourself worrying a great deal or feel fearful about carrying out your duties to your satisfaction.

4. By listening to others, it is sometimes possible to discover something you had been unaware of—something you can improve upon—or it may be possible to reach a compromise.

5. Not all issues can be easily resolved. You may need to seek confidential advice from somebody who knows and understands the medical context well—a representative of an organization supporting IMGs (some are listed at the end of this chapter) or from a professional organization like the British Medical Association (BMA). Some NHS organizations offer mediation through the medical staffing or Human Resources (HR) department.

The GMC now has web pages advising doctors of all levels of seniority how to deal with racism and discrimination (experienced or witnessed), as well as how to reduce the effects of bias.[31,32]

Summary

We have focused here on the needs of IMGs—not only for the sake of the individuals themselves but also because we have growing numbers of IMGs upon whose care we rely in the UK. We owe it to our IMGs to make their journey easier. But as we have discussed in the latter part of the chapter, that journey is anything but easy.

We started by considering our five career-planning stages, suggesting that IMGs use the model more iteratively given their greater breadth of experience at home and in an adopted country. We went on to outline an 'anatomy' of UK training and careers. We looked at the portfolio route—an increasingly common way to have one's experience and expertise recognized. We considered the specific needs of refugee doctors.

If there is a common thread running through all of this, we would say it is having the courage and patience to reach out for support. Doing so can help with the really difficult issues—like the differential attainment gap and the differential referral gap. The differential attainment gap is the lesser likelihood of achieving a pass in an exam if you are 'ethnic' in origin. The differential referral gap is the greater likelihood of doctors of 'ethnic' origin being referred to the medical regulator. There is now greater recognition that with greater understanding, small issues should not spiral out of proportion. The GMC-commissioned review reminds us that when we feel supported as individuals, we can grow and develop.

References

1. **General Medical Council** (2022). *The state of medical education and practice in the UK: the workforce report.* https://www.gmc-uk.org/-/media/documents/workforce-report-2022---full-report_pdf-94540077.pdf

2. **Medical Schools Council** (2021). *Medical Schools Council position statement.* https://www.medschools.ac.uk/media/2899/the-expansion-of-medical-student-numbers-in-the-united-kingdom-msc-position-paper-october-2021.pdf

3. **Saluja, S., Rudolfson, N., … & Shrime, M.G.** (2020). The impact of physician migration on mortality in low and middle-income countries: an economic modelling study. *BMJ Global Health.* 5(1):e001535. DOI: 10.1136/bmjgh-2019-001535

4. **Carr, A.** (2021). OET vs IELTS: Finding the most appropriate way to test language skills for medicine. *ESP Today.* 9(1):89–106. DOI: org/10.18485/esptoday.2021.9.1.5Carr, 2021).

5. **General Medical Council** (2023). *Unlocking the potential of the SAS workforce.* https://www.gmc-uk.org/news/news-archive/unlocking-the-potential-of-the-sas-workforce

6. **General Medical Council** (2024). *Good medical practice.* https://www.gmc-uk.org/ethical-guidance/ethical-guidance-for-doctors/good-medical-practice

7. **General Medical Council** (n.d.). *Working as a GP in the UK.* https://www.gmc-uk.org/registration-and-licensing/the-medical-register/a-guide-to-the-medical-register/gp-registration/working-as-a-gp-in-the-uk

8. **Owen, K., Hopkins, T., … & Dale, J.** (2019). GP retention in the UK: a worsening crisis. Findings from a cross-sectional survey. *BMJ Open.* 9(2):e026048. DOI: 10.1136/bmjopen-2018-026048

9. **Allaboudy, M., Ali, A., & Masud, T.** (2018). Gaining a certificate of eligibility for specialist registration (CESR) in the UK. *QJM.* **111**(suppl. 1):hcy200–068. https://doi.org/10.1093/qjmed/hcy200.068

10. **Health Education England & NHS Improvement** (2019, February). Maximising the potential: essential measures to support SAS doctors. https://www.hee.nhs.uk/sites/defa ult/files/documents/SAS_Report_Web.pdf

11. **Ong, Y.L., & Gayen, A.** (2003). Helping refugee doctors get their first jobs: the pan-London clinical attachment scheme. *Hosp Med.* **64**(8):488–490. DOI: 10.12968/hosp.2003.64.8.2265

12. **Piętka-Nykaza, E.** (2015). 'I want to do anything which is decent and relates to my profession': refugee doctors' and teachers' strategies of re-entering their professions in the UK. *J Refug Stud.* **28**(4):523–543. https://doi.org/10.1093/jrs/fev008

13. **MacKenzie Davey, K., & Jones, C.** (2020). Refugees' narratives of career barriers and professional identity. *Career Dev Int.* **25**(1):49–66. https://doi.org/10.1108/CDI-12-2018-0315

14. **Shah, R., Moodambail, A., … & Mulamehic, F.** (2021). An evaluation of the CAPS refugee doctor scheme in London—a survey of outcomes. *Educ Prim Care.* **32**(2):100–103. DOI:10.1080/14739879.2020.1857662

15. **Richardson, J.T.** (2008). *Degree attainment, ethnicity and gender: a literature review.* https://oro.open.ac.uk/11535/1/11535.pdf

16. **Woolf, K., Potts, H.W., & McManus, I.C.** (2011). Ethnicity and academic performance in UK trained doctors and medical students: systematic review and meta-analysis. *BMJ.* **342**:d901. DOI: 10.1136/bmj.d901

17. **McManus, I.C., & Wakeford, R.** (2014). PLAB and UK graduates' performance on MRCP (UK) and MRCGP examinations: data linkage study. *BMJ.* **348**:g2621. https://doi.org/10.1136/BMJ.g2621

18. British Association of Physicians of Indian Origin (2014). CSA judicial review. https://www.bapio.co.uk/csa-judicial-review/

19. **Tiffin, P.A., & Paton, L.W.** (2021). Differential attainment in the MRCPsych according to ethnicity and place of qualification between 2013 and 2018: a UK cohort study. *PMJ.* **97**(1154):764–776. DOI. 10.1136/postgradmedj-2020-137913

20. **Woolf, K., Rich, A., … & Griffin, A.** (2016). Perceived causes of differential attainment in UK postgraduate medical training: a national qualitative study. *BMJ Open.* **6**(11):e013429.

21. **Slowther, A., Lewando Hundt, G.A., … & Taylor, R.** (2012). Experiences of non-UK-qualified doctors working within the UK regulatory framework: a qualitative study. *JRSM.* **105**(4):157–165. DOI 10.1258/jrsm.2011.110256.

22. **Khan, F.A., Chikkatagaiah, S., … & Kingston, P.** (2015). International medical graduates (IMGs) in the UK—a systematic review of their acculturation and adaptation. *J Int Migr Integr.* **16**:743–759. DOI 10.1007/s12134-014-0368-y.

23. **Jalal, M., Bardhan, K.D., … & Illing, J.** (2019). Overseas doctors of the NHS: migration, transition, challenges and towards resolution. *Future Healthc J.* **6**(1):76–81. https://doi.org/10.7861/futurehosp.6-1-76

24. **Roe, V., Patterson, F., … & Edwards, H.** (2019). *What supported your success in training?. A qualitative exploration of the factors associated with an absence of an ethnic attainment gap in post-graduate specialty training.* GMC. https://www.gmc-uk.org/-/media/docume nts/gmc-da-final-report-success-factors-in-training-211119_pdf-80914221.pdf

25. **Chukwudi, I.** (2022). UKFPO F2 Standalone: a brief guide. *Ann Med Surg.* **82**:104594. DOI: 10.1016/j.amsu.2022.104594

26. **Esmail, A., & Everington, S.** (1994). General Medical Council. Complaints may reflect racism. *BMJ.* **308**(6940):1374.

27. **Humphrey, C., Hickman, S., & Gulliford, M. C.** (2011). Place of medical qualification and outcomes of UK General Medical Council 'fitness to practise' process: cohort study. *BMJ.* 342:1374. https://doi.org/10.1136/bmj.d1817

28. **Mahase, E.** (2022). GMC to review Manjula Arora case after backlash from doctors. *BMJ.* **377**:o1350. https://doi.org/10.1136/bmj.o1350

29. **General Medical Council** (2022). *The GMC's handling of the case of Dr Manjula Arora: An independent learning review.* https://www.gmc-uk.org/-/media/documents/the-gmc-s-handling-of-the-case-of-dr-manjula-arora-an-independent-learning-review-professor-94950326.pdf

30. **General Medical Council** (2019). *Fair to Refer? Reducing disproportionality in fitness to practice concerns reported to the GMC.* https://www.gmc-uk.org/-/media/documents/fair-to-refer-report_pdf-79011677.pdf

31. **General Medical Council** (2024). *Racism in the workplace.* https://www.gmc-uk.org/ethical-guidance/ethical-hub/racism-in-the-workplace

32. **General Medical Council** (2022). *Speaking up.* https://www.gmc-uk.org/ethical-guidance/ethical-hub/speaking-up

Further reading

Hodkinson, J., & Lok, P. (2022). NHS launches first standardised induction programme for international medical graduates. *BMJ.* **378**:o1624. https://doi.org/10.1136/bmj.o1624

Nageswaran, P., & Chakravorty, I. (2022). Dignity at work standards: proceedings from a consensus summit. *The Physician.* **7**(3):1–4. doi.org/10.38192/1.7.3.12

Further information

Association of Pakistani Physicians of Northern Europe (APPNE) https://www.appne.uk/

Black Medical Society https://www.blackmedicalsociety.co.uk/

BMJ Careers https://www.bmj.com/careers/article/a-guide-to-img-applications-for-specialty-training-in-the-uk

The Bridges Programmes https://bridgesprogrammes.org.uk/

British Association of Physicians of Indian Origin (BAPIO) https://www.bapio.co.uk/

British International Doctors Association (BIDA) https://www.bidaonline.co.uk/

British Islamic Medical Association https://britishima.org/

General Medical Council (GMC) https://www.gmc-uk.org

GMC: Help for Refugee Doctors https://www.gmc-uk.org/registration-and-licensing/join-the-register/before-you-apply/help-for-refugee-doctors

GMC: Specialty specific guidance for portfolio pathway applications https://www.gmc-uk.org/registration-and-licensing/join-the-register/registration-applications/specialty-specific-guidance-for-cesr-and-cegpr

GMC: Tackling Differential Attainment https://www.gmc-uk.org/education/standards-guidance-and-curricula/guidance/tackling-differential-attainment

Medical Training Initiative http://www.aomrc.org.uk/medical-training-initiative

Melanin Medics https://www.melaninmedics.com/

Muslim Doctors Association https://muslimdoctors.org/

NHS Employers https://www.nhsemployers.org/

NHS Information for Overseas Doctors https://www.healthcareers.nhs.uk/explore-roles/doctors/information-overseas-doctors

One2one mentoring network for black and minority ethnic professionals https://one2onementoring.com/

REACHE Northwest of England https://www.reache.org.uk/

Refugee Action https://www.refugee-action.org.uk/

Refugee Assessment and Guidance Unit https://londonmet.ac.uk/services-and-facilities/refugee-assessment-and-guidance-unit/

Society of Chinese Medical Practitioners UK http://scmp-uk.org/

UK Foundation Programme https://foundationprogramme.nhs.uk

Wales Asylum Seeker and Refugee Doctors Group https://www.dpia.org.uk/projects/ward/

Chapter 8

Congratulations or commiserations

This chapter focuses on the question of 'What next?'—something that you'll ask yourself once you've received a definitive response to your application. We start with the perhaps unexpected topic of learning from success before moving on to more familiar territory—what to do if the response is not what you'd hoped for. This is an important, yet often overlooked topic in career planning. While there will always be some rare individuals whose progress seems unstoppable—the majority of us (by definition) are closer to average. This means career setbacks can occur along the way. Fortunately, there are psychological approaches that can help—to which we have added some of the practical tips that have emerged from our work supporting doctors. At the end of the day your perseverance is likely to be rewarded because ultimately the world always needs doctors.

Learning from success

It makes sense to learn from our positive experiences as well as from the negative ones, but many of us were brought up to think of feeling proud as an inappropriate indulgence. Whether or not that is the case, we want to argue that doctors can learn from positive performance in the same way that sportspeople do. The power of 'Marginal Gains' was made popular by David Brailsford, the GB cycling team coach as the team prepared for the 2008 and 2012 Olympics. The approach seems to involve considering *every*thing that could conceivably affect performance from the structure of the bike, the kit, the massage gels, the beds, pillows, even the cyclists' sleep positions. Nothing is off limits—including what went well, and how to improve still further. So the purpose of a comprehensive review of success is to identify approaches you want to retain in future, as well as things you can do to improve further.

You won't necessarily have video footage of your performance to hand, but you will have the ability to reflect on your success. Aiming to capture the essentials of your performance before they recede into distant memory, we offer (in Box 8.1) some suggestions. If you have a recent successful application to review, thinking and ideally writing down your responses to the prompts will start a process of preparing for further future successes.

If your application was unsuccessful

It seems more natural to want to learn from scenarios that *don't* go as planned. But this may be a bigger ask as doing so is, of course, emotionally harder. The strength of your feelings will vary according to your circumstances, your financial position, and how

> ## Box 8.1 **Reviewing your success**
>
> ### Your preparation
>
> - It's often said that preparation is key. Was this the case for you? How *did* you prepare?
> - If a person who was preparing for a similar challenge asked you to advise, what preparation would you suggest?
>
> ### Your written application and its supporting documents
>
> - How would you describe the approach you took to applying?
> - What do you think the selection panel liked about your application?
> - What do *you* like about the application you submitted?
> - How do you feel you dealt with your areas of relative weakness? Were you able to mitigate these or compensate for them by showcasing your strengths?
> - Would you deal with your relative weaknesses the same or differently next time?
>
> ### Your exam/interview elements
>
> - What went well in the exam and interview scenarios?
> - How did your preparation help you with the scenarios?
> - Did everything happen as expected? If you needed to think on your feet, what helped you to do so?
> - How did you manage nerves or over-confidence?
>
> ### Overall
>
> - What would you most like to be able to repeat for similar occasions in future?
> - What could you do to further improve your performance?

much you felt you really *needed* that particular post. Your feelings will be influenced by your prior experience of success and failure. Experiencing failure for the first time can be surprisingly stressful. Many successful people's self-esteem seems to depend on succeeding at *everything* they try.

We offer the following prompts to help you manage your inevitable feelings of disappointment.

- When you learnt to walk in infancy, how many times might you have fallen? Given the high number it's likely to be, it's fortunate that you wouldn't have had the cognitive capacity to over-think the situation.

- Through what formative experiences in childhood or adulthood did you learn your particular emotional responses to success and failure?

- What do you hope your children, nephews, nieces, or friends' children will learn about the meaning of success and failure?

- If failure were a skill, what would it involve doing (or thinking)?

Our stress responses and ways of coping differ, yet we can all benefit from some of the tried and tested methods to enhance our coping. We discuss in Box 8.2 what stress is and some of the distinct coping strategies, including growth mindset (Figure 8.1).

Growth mindset in practice

In light of mindset theory, we want to encourage you to consider:

- When you receive negative feedback, what do you find yourself thinking and feeling? What would it take for you to see negative feedback as an opportunity?

- How do you think your particular mindset beliefs developed? Can you think of any formative experiences in childhood or adulthood that may have contributed?

- In order to develop growth mindset, what fundamental beliefs might you need to let go of?

- Who might you regard as good growth mindset role models? (a role model being a person you consider 'like me', who you'd like to emulate).

We now want to encourage you to consider how growth mindset could be applied to a recent unsuccessful application. If you don't have an unsuccessful application to hand, you could adapt the questions in Box 8.3 to *any* occasion or occasions in which you performed sub-optimally. A good starting point is first to identify the kinds of errors you made or the errors you tend to make—which when corrected will enhance your performance. It is worth keeping in mind that although growth mindset is about learning from failure, its aim is to enhance performance.

Seeking feedback

An important aspect of growth mindset is both seeking feedback and responding to it. Feedback is important because it can be hard to accurately assess our own performance. We often have personal blind spots. Consider, for example, the Dunning–Kruger effect, well known to medical educators (Box 8.4).

Turning to the applied research, it shouldn't surprise us to know that high quality feedback brings about positive emotional states for unsuccessful job seekers—who then feel more motivated in continuing with job applications.[1] To count as high quality, feedback needs to be sufficiently detailed. Unfortunately, poor quality feedback can be de-motivating, particularly for those already struggling with confidence as it can leave people feeling that they don't know the specific things that they need to change, to improve their performance.

In considering your own application, if feedback is available upon request, it makes sense to request it. But if you find the feedback to be superficial or limited to rankings, you could improve its quality by discussing your application with a trusted person— ideally someone senior who knows your work and who understands the recruitment

We owe much of our understanding of coping to psychologists Richard Lazarus and his student Susan Folkman.[2] In their transactional theory of stress and coping they posited something that now seems like common sense: that as humans we constantly appraise and re-appraise the situations we encounter.

When situations are appraised as threatening or harmful, we recruit strategies to cope. Our coping strategies may be oriented to helping us solve the problem itself, or they maybe help us manage the emotions thrown up. Some coping strategies are more effective than others. 'Stress' occurs when an event is appraised as threatening or harmful *and* as exceeding our capacity to cope. Stress is associated with physiological markers, the best-known of which is raised cortisol.

Doctors, as we discuss in Chapter 12, can experience considerable anxiety and depression so it's surprising that more studies of doctors' coping have not been published. When active coping strategies such as problem-solving or seeking social support are used, doctors tend to experience fewer mental health symptoms. In contrast, strategies that include self-blame, wishing things were different, and avoiding thinking about the topic are associated with feeling anxious or depressed.[3,4] It is possible that doctors' coping is influenced by the culture within UK medicine with its tendency to emphasize appearing rational and invulnerable.[5–7]

A promising development in psychology is *growth mindset* theory.[8] This is a theory focusing on the ideas we hold about our own intellect and abilities. At one end of the scale we might believe that intellectual ability is fluid and can grow (growth mindset). At the other, we may believe these attributes to be inherited and fixed (fixed mindset). We can, of course, occupy a middle position. For child and adult learners, believing in the potential for growth is itself associated with growth in actual attainment—a self-fulfilling prophesy. Our mindset appears to predict our response to setbacks when they occur. Those with a growth mindset respond with greater striving than those with fixed mindsets who are more inclined to avoid taking risks. Those with fixed mindset place greater value on appearing to be competent over monitoring their actual learning—perhaps reproducing some of the cultural norms common within the medical profession.

Fortunately it's possible to develop a growth mindset—to learn how to think of failures as learning opportunities. 'Mindset interventions' are surprisingly simple and effective, having been trialled in schools and colleges around the world. Learners are taught to think of the mind as having muscle-like qualities, needing practice. Less work has been carried out in work contexts and still less within healthcare. However there is some indication that those with growth mindsets may be more engaged, may experience greater job satisfaction and tend to perform better than people with fixed mindsets.[9] One study used a neonatal resuscitation computer game simulation to demonstrate that health professionals high in growth mindset made fewer errors than their fixed mindset colleagues.[10]

In the absence of further research we can't know for sure how medical students and doctors might benefit from mindset interventions. They might be ideal students of mindset, knowledgeable as they are about our brains' plasticity. To fully embrace mindset theory, medical educators would perhaps need to let go of some of the more traditional practices such as ranking and categorizing learners which can inadvertently convey a message that potential is fixed.

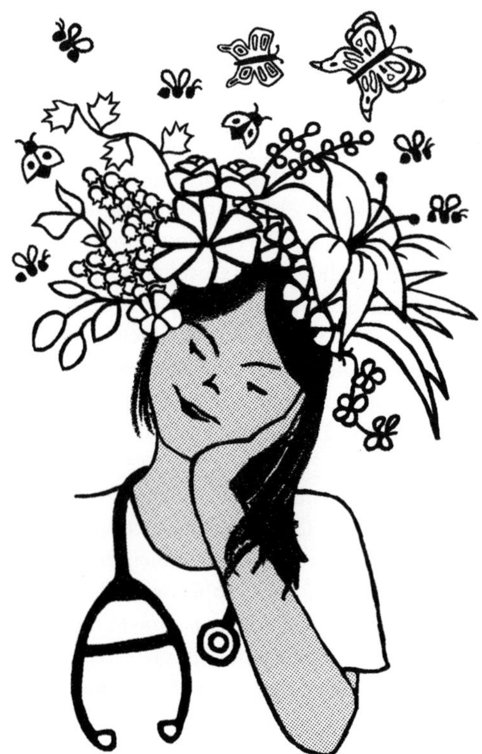

Figure 8.1 Growth mindset.

process. Given how biased we can all be, it's useful to gain more than one opinion. And to increase the chance that the conversation will be productive it's worth preparing some questions in advance.

Next steps towards successful application

Hopefully, you'll arrive at an action plan that's specific, achievable, and timed, thus increasing your chance of submitting an improved application. You might plan, for example:

◆ to apply for a number of different positions;

◆ to re-apply for the same position as well as alternative positions as back-ups;

◆ to build up additional experience: taster days, presentations, teaching sessions, etc.;

◆ to arrange a mock interview with feedback.

Box 8.3 **Reviewing an unsuccessful application**

Preparation

- How did you prepare for the application that was not successful?
- How would you like to prepare differently next time?
- How much time would you need for this?
- How would you ideally like to you use this time?
- Who could help you? How?

Written application elements—the form, uploaded 'evidence'

- What was your approach to the selection process?
- How could you adjust your approach?
- What do you think the selection panel liked most about your application?
- What do you think they didn't like?
- What did *you* like most about the approach you took and about your application itself?
- What didn't you like?

Exam/interview elements

- What went well? What went less well?
- Did things go as expected? Did anything happen that was unexpected?
- What topics did you handle best and least well? What's your theory as to why the difficult topics were difficult for you?
- What formats did you struggle with the most? What's your theory about why these formats were hard for you?
- What effects, if any, did anxiety or over-confidence have? If relevant, what could you do to reduce their impact?
- How might you change or adapt your approach next time?

Should I appeal a decision that seems wrong?

You may feel you have grounds to appeal against the outcome of your application. There will be an appeal policy which should tell you whether or not you are eligible to appeal. It's worth reading the criteria for appeal carefully and talking the matter

Box 8.4 **The Dunning–Kruger effect**

The Dunning–Kruger effect is a consistent finding seen in numerous experiments.

It is sometimes called meta-ignorance because it refers to the ways in which we don't know what we don't know. In a nutshell, we are surprisingly inaccurate in our estimates of our performance and we're particularly inaccurate when our performance is well below average.

In one experiment, students taking a test were asked to estimate their scores. Figure 8.2 shows the students' estimated scores along with their actual scores. Impossibly, most students rated themselves above average. Similar biases occur across a range of skills studied—including doctors rating their ability to perform various procedures and drivers rating their driving ability.[11,12] An interesting twist is that the skilled performers slightly *under*-estimate their performance. It is suggested that highly skilled performers may not realize how much less skilled other people than they are.[13]

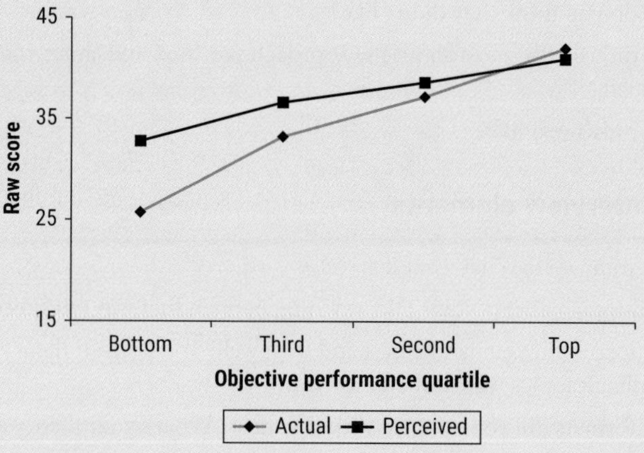

Figure 8.2 Actual and self-rated test scores.

Reprinted from *Advances in Experimental Social Psychology*, 44, Dunning D, 'The Dunning–Kruger effect: On being ignorant of one's own ignorance', pp. 247-296, Copyright 2011, with permission from Elsevier. Adapted from Dunning D, et al., Why people fail to recognize their own competence. *Current Directions in Psychological Science*, 12, 3, pp. 83-87. Copyright © 2003 by Association for Psychological Science. Reprinted by Permission of Sage Publications

through with a senior colleague. It's certainly not the case that it is *never* worth appealing. However, you need to weigh up how much time and effort (including the emotional work) an appeal might entail. There is also the question as to whether appealing might unhelpfully cause you to put everything on hold rather than moving on and embracing what you need to do next.

The case study in Box 8.5 aims to show how some of the principles in the foregoing discussion can play out in practice.

Box 8.5 **A common problem**

Sam's application for surgery was an afterthought, so she was not surprised when her application was unsuccessful. Previously Sam had experienced great uncertainty about what to do. When Sam mentioned to her consultant that she was considering applying for surgical training, she was asked how driven she really was. It seemed obvious that she hadn't demonstrated a passion for surgery in her F1 post. It was only now, as a consequence of emergency department (ED) work in F2 that Sam realized the pleasure she experienced in carrying out procedures. Unfortunately during the COVID-19 pandemic, Sam's surgical post in her F2 year had not allowed Sam to gain the level of experience it might otherwise have had. It was hard to leave the ward to attend theatre. When she did manage to gain access, she made a 'nuisance' of herself, asking questions and offering to assist. Sometimes Sam's offers were taken up but this was not invariable and sometimes Sam really did feel that she was an annoyance to her seniors in theatre.

Sam had clocked up a considerable amount of experience carrying out quality improvement projects during her FY years. But the projects were in areas that were considered not to be sufficiently relevant to surgery. Sam also struggled to demonstrate *commitment to the specialty* which was disheartening.

Luckily Sam found a senior surgical trainee willing to give her feedback on her application and she realized that the problem wasn't personal. It was a common case of not having had enough opportunity to gain the experience required for a high quality application to surgical training. Sam's action plan now included: (1) gaining more surgical experience as a clinical fellow—to fill most or all of the gaps; (2) teaching medical students (and anybody else willing to be taught); (3) participating in QI projects on surgical topics; and (4) finding a mentor to help her find and take opportunities, to check out her portfolio and help identify the best way to communicate commitment to the specialty.

Taking consolation from today's variety of career shapes

Sam's case involved taking extra time and being prepared to repeat some of the more important experiences. Doing so can feel immensely frustrating. It can also be anxiety-provoking to find you're not first off the block in the career race. But really, should a satisfying career be a race at all? This is perhaps one area in which doctors and athletes' careers differ.

Career researchers have come to think of the traditional progression from the bottom to the top of an organization as less common than it once was. Described by Douglas Hall in his 1976 book *Careers in Organizations*,[14] the Protean career was conceived as a different way of understanding careers (Box 8.6).

You might think that the Protean Career Orientation has a corporate feel to it. If so, how could it be relevant to doctors? We would argue that in medicine, we are

> ### Box 8.6 **Protean careers**
>
> Douglas Hall observed that careers had become more changeable in the sense of being driven more by the person than by the employing organization. The name Protean, derives from the Greek god who changed his shape at will.
>
> Protean Career Orientation (PCO) has been widely studied, conceptualized as people's sense of their need for freedom, growth, and well-being. PCO is found to be associated with job satisfaction, organizational commitment, choosing work–life balance and with subjective (though not objective) measures of career success.[15]
>
> One problem though, is the circularity of the reasoning: those with a protean orientation may become more satisfied with their careers on account of their protean attitudes. Even if this is the case, it is still heartening that PCO does not bring about detrimental outcomes.

now less inclined to think of a job as a job for life. Younger doctors appear to think in more protean ways, causing workforce planners to have to think more flexibly. The percentage of doctors choosing to take a post-foundation training break (F3 year) increased almost threefold to 65% in 2019[16] and may continue to increase further. The list of reasons for doctors making this choice includes their wish to take some control over their careers while also improving their work–life balance. So the idea of varying career shapes has gained traction in medicine.

With the aid of a case study (Box 8.7), we can consider what a Protean Medical Career Orientation might look like.

An acceptance and commitment approach

Acceptance and commitment therapy (ACT) is a third wave approach to CBT (cognitive behavioural therapy). Acceptance is about tackling mental experiences—thoughts, feelings, and conundrums in a way that is less judgemental than is usual. Even if you can't change the past, the reasoning goes, you can wonder if your way of coping is helping you progress with the life you want to lead. Knowing about the life you want to lead—your values—is the 'commitment' part. 'Acceptance and commitment' is not about being passive nor is it about giving up. It is more a case of getting to grips with situations that arise.[17]

We are not suggesting that everybody who doesn't succeed should jump into therapy and neither of us are ACT therapists. However we find the principles of this approach resonate with our own values and we offer the following prompts as an aid to dealing with any lack of success you may encounter in your career:

◆ If you have been unsuccessful, what do you think the reasons may be?—some may reflect your approach, others may reflect the way the system works—or luck.

◆ What are the most important parts of your plan? Why are they important to you?

◆ Who can help you to achieve your plan?

- How many times do you want to apply for this particular type of post?
- What offers are within your reach?
- What back-up plans interest you? How consistent are they with your values?
- What do you want to do next?
- How are you coping? Is this helping? How can you pace yourself?

Box 8.7 Adam's contingency planning

Wanting to be engaging with the 'big picture stuff' in his career, Adam planned a career in public health. A particular interest of Adam's was forecasting future health needs. But Adam struggled with multitasking. He had suffered from an autoimmune condition as well as depression as a medical student, but he had learnt to manage these issues and went on to have some great experiences in medical school. He counted his intercalated BSc as a period in which he had undergone considerable self-development.

Adam was unsuccessful in his public health application. He'd done well but hadn't scored highly enough as the competition had been intense. Another specialty that attracted Adam was virology. He realized that the training path would be very different. Adam didn't mind the prospect of two years in internal medicine, but he worried that the focus in virology might be too narrow given his broad interest in healthcare.

Adam arranged to meet up with his BSc supervisor. At the time of his BSc, it hadn't been possible to get a publication as his project had been part of a larger one which hadn't progressed at the expected rate. The larger project was now going much better and a paper was a possibility although Adam's data would need to be re-analysed. If Adam took this on, he should be able to present the work at a conference. Adam was keen to re-kindle his interest but needed to create the time to devote to the project. He signed up with the hospital bank and began looking for a clinical fellowship to give him more flexibility in his F3 year.

Adam also made a contingency plan—to put in the best public health application he could and at the same time apply to IMT core training. He would tailor his experience to the requirements of each specialty. An offer came in for IMT, which Adam 'held' until he'd heard back from public health. Unfortunately, second time round he was still unsuccessful as his project hadn't progressed quickly enough to benefit his application. Adam was not as devastated as he thought he'd be. In the aftermath of the COVID-19 pandemic, virology now seemed critically important to Adam and the contact he was having with the lab stimulated a new interest in lab-based research. Adam reconciled himself to a patient-facing training. He took steps to manage his own health and also looked into the option of going down an academic route.

Summary

In this chapter we started with how one can best pick oneself up after a setback. But we have also included learning from success. Some wonderful 'virtuous circles' can arise when you do so. It's possible that most of us don't allow sufficient time to reflect on the points of our career when everything has gone according to plan.

In relation to setbacks, we drew upon the psychology of coping and of growth mindset arguing that these approaches can be helpful for doctors. You may have noticed how much overlap exists in the psychological theories we draw upon. 'Acceptance' is conceptually similar to 'growth mindset'. Or perhaps they are two sides of one coin. Both give the appearance of being common sense but this can happen with robust psychological research.

In our work with doctors, we find that when good psychology can be brought to bear on career planning, a feeling of liberation may follow. Unless we're highly unusual and lucky, we are all likely to experience *both* success and failure throughout our careers—as well as in our lives beyond work. The ability to adapt to challenge is an important one to embrace.

References

1. **Chawla, N., Gabriel, A.S.,** ... **& Slaughter, J.E.** (2019). Does feedback matter for job search self-regulation? It depends on feedback quality. *Personnel Psychol.* **72**(4):513–541. DOI: 10.1111/peps.12320

2. **Lazarus, R.S., & Folkman, S.** (1987). Transactional theory and research on emotions and coping. *Eur J Pers.* **1**(3):141–169. DOI: org/10.1002/per.2410010304

3. **Firth-Cozens, J., & Morrison, L.A.** (1989). Sources of stress and ways of coping in junior house officers. *Stress Med.* **5**(2):121–126. https://doi.org/10.1002/smi.2460050210

4. **Tattersall, A.J., Bennett, P., & Pugh, S.** (1999). Stress and coping in hospital doctors. *Stress Medicine, 15*(2), 109–113.

5. **Lyons, B., Gibson, M., & Dolezal, L.** (2018). Stories of shame. *Lancet.* **391**(10130):1568–1569. DOI: 10.1016/S0140-6736(18)30897-3.

6. **Elton, C.** (2018). *Also human: the inner lives of doctors.* William Heinemann.

7. **Riley, R., Buszewicz, M.,** ... **& Chew-Graham, C.** (2021). Sources of work-related psychological distress experienced by UK-wide foundation and junior doctors: a qualitative study. *BMJ Open.* **11**(6):e043521. DOI:10.1136/bmjopen-2020-043521

8. **Yeager, D S., & Dweck, C.S.** (2020). What can be learned from growth mindset controversies? *Am Psychol.* **75**(9):1269 –1284. https://doi.org/10.1037/amp0000794

9. **Han, S.J., & Stieha, V.** (2020). Growth mindset for human resource development: A scoping review of the literature with recommended interventions. *Hum Resour Dev Rev.* **19**(3):309–331. DOI: 10.1177/1534484320939739

10. **Cutumisu, M., Brown, M.R.,** ... **& Schmölzer, G. M.** (2018). Growth mindset moderates the effect of the neonatal resuscitation program on performance in a computer-based game training simulation. *Front Pediatr.* **6**:195. https://doi.org/10.3389/fped.2018.00195

11. **Barnsley, L., Lyon, P. M.,** ... **& Field, M.J.** (2004). Clinical skills in junior medical officers: a comparison of self-reported confidence and observed competence. *Med Educ.* **38**(4):358–367.

12. **Vnuk, A., Owen, H., & Plummer, J.** (2006). Assessing proficiency in adult basic life support: student and expert assessment and the impact of video recording. *Med* Teach. **28**(5):429–434. DOI: 10.1080/01421590600625205

13. **Dunning, D.** (2011). The Dunning–Kruger effect: on being ignorant of one's own ignorance. In: Dunning, D., ed. *Advances in experimental social psychology.* Academic Press; Vol. **44**; 247–296. https://doi.org/10.1016/B978-0-12-385522-0.00005-6

14. **Hall, D.T.** (1996). Protean careers of the 21st century. *Acad Manag Perspect.* **10**(4):8–16. https://doi.org/10.5465/ame.1996.3145315

15. **Hall, D.T., Yip, J., & Doiron, K.** (2018). Protean careers at work: self-direction and values orientation in psychological success. *Ann Rev Organ Psychol Organ Behav.* **5**:129–156. https://doi.org/10.1146/annurev-orgpsych-032117-104631

16. **Silverton, R., & Freeth, D.** (2022). *The F3 phenomenon: exploring a new norm and its implications.* Health Education England.

17. **Harris, R.** (2006). Embracing your demons: an overview of acceptance and commitment therapy. *Psychother Aus.* **12**(4):70–76.

Further reading

Dweck, C.S. (2017). *Mindset.* Robinson.

Halstead, L. (2021). *Becoming a true athlete: a practical philosophy for flourishing through sport.* Sequoia Books.

Harris, R. (2010). *The confidence gap: from fear to freedom.* Robinson.

Harris, R (2021). *When life hits hard: how to transcend grief, crisis, and loss with acceptance and commitment therapy.* New Harbinger Publications.

Further information

CREST forms (Certificate of Readiness to Enter Specialty Training) https://medical.hee.nhs.uk/medical-training-recruitment/medical specialty-training/foundation-competencies/certificate-of-readiness/crest

Working with ACT https://workingwithact.com

Part II

Challenges along the way

Chapter 9

What if I'm not drawn to any specialty?

We want to spend some time considering the small but significant number of doctors for whom no specialty seems right. Such a realization can form gradually, occasionally starting as early as medical school. Whatever the stage however, the experience can be unnerving as there is still a taboo around the idea of 'giving up' medicine. In contrast, we will argue that any sense of career unease should be taken seriously. Decisions about one's career are among the biggest decisions we take in our lives so a lingering sense of career dissatisfaction should not be overlooked.

We start by discussing how many doctors don't want to continue practising in a traditional way. We go on to discuss career regret and some of the issues that face doctors looking to change career and we outline how to use our staged model in this situation. Whether you're choosing between the traditional medical specialties or looking more widely, the structured approach is the same.

Doctors who no longer want to doctor

The UK Medical Careers Research Group routinely ask doctors about their career plans. The group's surveys show the number of doctors considering leaving medicine increased from 4% in 1999 to 9.6% in 2015.[1,2] The number who *actually* leave is harder to know. We do know that the proportion of doctors relinquishing their licences to practice was 3.45% in 2021 and 3.8% in 2022.[3] These figures may not accurately reflect the numbers leaving because some leavers retain their licence, at least for a period. Asked for their reasons for considering leaving, 476 doctors sampled by the UK Medical Career Research Group indicated the following (Figure 9.1)[2]. It may seem surprising that concerns about the culture, state of the NHS, or policies have been uppermost for so long. We might conclude that some things never change!

An alternative approach is to survey doctors who have actually given up their practice. *Completing the Picture* was one such survey commissioned by the General Medical Council (GMC), directed at doctors no longer practising in the UK.[4] The heterogeneous group of 13,158 doctors, whose average age was 45 years, included those working abroad, those not practising at all, and retired doctors. Most commonly, the doctors cited their dissatisfaction with 'the role, place of work or NHS culture' (36%). 'Burnout or work-related stress' was cited by 27%. Others' decisions had been influenced by life cycle issues— returning to a country of previous residence, moving to support a partner, or retirement.

Completing the Picture echoes the findings of an American survey in which 1,576 pre-retirement age 'medically inactive' physicians responded.[5] Thirty-eight per cent of the physicians cited 'personal and health concerns' while 22% had been professionally dissatisfied.

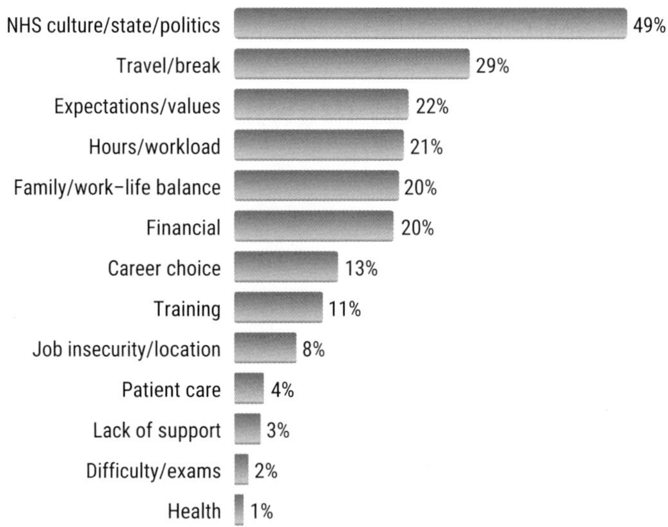

Figure 9.1 Why UK doctors considered leaving circa 2015.
Data from Lambert, T.W., Smith, F., & Goldacre, M.J. (2018). Why doctors consider leaving UK medicine: qualitative analysis of comments from questionnaire surveys three years after graduation. *Journal of the Royal Society of Medicine*, 111(1), 18-30. Table 2, p 24. DOI: 10.1177/0141076817738502

But the larger scale surveys can only provide broad categories of experience and their respondents tend to be older. Smaller, qualitative studies are therefore helpful in supplementing their findings, giving a more nuanced picture. Pathmanathan and Snelling[6] interviewed a sample of 17 doctors recruited using social media. The sample included junior doctors, GPs, and consultants who had left the profession the year before the outbreak of Covid. Many spoke of a lack of congruence between their own values and those of the healthcare system in which they worked. Some felt thwarted in their ability to deliver patient care, experiencing a lack of autonomy. Doctors spoke of the deleterious effects of their work on their personal and family lives.

It is possible that the after-effects of the pandemic will further affect the number of doctors choosing to leave the profession. Our reason for discussing a number of studies here is that we believe the stigma of considering leaving the profession—and of actually leaving—is such that doctors may overlook the available information. Yet it is important for those considering leaving to know that others have followed the same path—and why.

Career regret

Regret is defined as the emotion we experience when realizing or imagining that our current situation would have been better, if only we had made different choices. It is an unpleasant emotional experience tinged with self-blame.[7] Career regret is surprisingly common. As many as 50% of a sample of 2,000 British pharmacists regretted their career choice.[8] In a group of British cardiac physiologists who regretted their career choice, the feeling of regret was associated with lower levels of job satisfaction and with comparing their own career unfavourably with those of other people.[9] But what about *doctors'* career regrets? Few studies are published. A US study followed medical students into their resident physician years.[10] As residents, 45% experienced symptoms of burnout while 14% experienced career regret. Unsurprisingly, burnout and career regret were correlated. Having experienced anxiety as a student predicted later burnout and career regret while the prior experience of feeling empathy as a student seemed to be protective. Career regret can fluctuate, depending on events at work—like feeling unsupported, feeling bullied, or struggling to progress. Events outside work can also accentuate career regret.

A related construct, the *Psychological Contract* has now become quite well-known. The psychological contract refers to an unwritten, subjective contract between the employer and the employee based upon the beliefs and expectations held by both parties.[11] The psychological contract can rather easily be experienced as having been breached, with associated feelings of anger, betrayal, or disappointment as well as effects on work performance and staff retention. A study of academic pharmacists' experiences of the psychological contract identified breaches in relation to workload, teaching load, pay progression, lack of support and facilities.[9]

A US study[12] followed new nursing and new accounting recruits who rated the job rewards they experienced as well as job costs, job satisfaction, and commitment in the year after starting in their job roles. Job reward is the experience of positivity, arising from the nature of the work, the pay, training opportunities, or promotion. Job costs are the unpleasant aspects of work—sometimes caused by work schedules or by the absence of rewards. The authors found that initially, the job costs experienced by the nurses and accountants did not seem to be important. Perhaps the new recruits expected to struggle a little. Over time however, the detrimental effects of job costs on the recruits' job commitment increased. For those who ultimately resigned their posts, the factor that was most influential was their perception of the quality of the available alternative job roles.

Identity change

Changes at work are sometimes likened to a process of grieving, the stages of which have been described by Elisabeth Kübler-Ross.[13] Denial may precede searching; feelings of depression can give way to acceptance. The stages don't necessarily occur 'in order'.[14] We consider grief a helpful metaphor given that a medical job is not 'just a job' but is typically a core part of a doctor's identity. Clare Gerada, former president of the Royal College of GPs suggests that the 'medical self-identity' may start to form early on—sometimes even before medical school entry.[15] As the medical identity may underly a sense of safety and belonging, it's not surprising that it would be hard to give up. Feelings of guilt and shame can easily occur, medicine tending to be seen as a 'noble' profession. Moreover, when a doctor indicates their intention to move on, it can be deeply unsettling for other people. Parents can be heavily invested in the fact of their daughter or son being a doctor, as can partners.

We think of identity formation and re-formation as a social process. As we will discuss, it is important to work around the taboo of leaving the profession in order to have the conversations that you need to have. Initially you may choose to talk confidentially with trusted supporters, as a way of getting used to talking about this sensitive issue.

Our case study in Box 9.1 illustrates the process of giving up one identity in favour of another.

Box 9.1 **Tessa in a world beyond medicine**

Tessa was as a highly conscientious medical student who was fascinated by the subject-matter. Finding visual topics like anatomy and biochemistry easy, she won prizes and commendations. But Tessa had to work hard to commit large volumes of facts to memory. At that time, final year clinical students frequently undertook student locum roles. For Tessa, doing so was unthinkable. Few of the realities of the medical role appealed. As the equivalent of an F1 doctor, Tessa enjoyed working with patients but worried about them as if they were members of her own family—which sometimes made it hard for her to think rationally. She always wanted the most experienced doctor's opinion, doubting she could be the right person to make a decision. With the stakes feeling this high, Tessa no longer found the subject-matter interesting.

Chemical pathology did appeal to Tessa with its more limited direct patient-contact. But when training in the specialty, the clinical responsibility once again weighed too heavily on Tessa who now considered moving into research or on to something non-medical. Then, quite suddenly, Tessa's boyfriend, Gavin, became ill with cancer, which he did not survive. Tessa took a period of leave to care for Gavin. To occupy her mind, Tessa learnt computer programming. As she began to programme, a eureka moment occurred, 'So *this* is how my brain works!'

Losing Gavin devasted Tessa. There was pressure to return to work soon after Gavin's death. Tessa asked if she might initially return to a non-clinical role. When this request was denied, she resigned. Tessa's contingency plan was to enrol on a computer science master's course as a mature student. Cutting her teeth in her first computer science job (building GP computer systems), Tessa experienced an overwhelming sense of wellbeing at work. For the first time, she was able to laugh and make friends at work! Work was no longer simply a matter of surviving. Tessa went on to work in computer programming and business analyst roles. She now works for a consultancy company as an IT project manager.

Along the way, Tessa was diagnosed with dyslexia. The diagnosis helped her understand her working memory difficulties (especially when stressed) and why she finds visual material easier to process. Nowadays, she can usually find work-arounds for these issues. Through practising self-compassion, Tessa is better able to reel herself in from over-conscientiousness. For Tessa, this was only possible when people's lives were no longer in her hands.

If you are contemplating a change—

◆ Could you imagine giving up your medical identity? If not, you might consider exploring the less-well-known medical specialities before contemplating leaving the profession.

◆ Most people talk to friends and family about work. It's worth considering which family members might understand your dilemmas. Which will struggle with their own feelings of disappointment?

◆ Would you consider talking to a professional helper like a coach or career counsellor?

◆ Do you perceive a psychological contract breach? If so, how would you describe it? The experience could help you work out your personal criteria for future work. Of course psychological contract breaches can occur in all sectors, so changing job role doesn't guarantee further breaches won't occur.

◆ Some people simply feel like a square peg in a round hole. They experience a mismatch between their own needs, talents, and interests on the one hand and the demands of the job on the other. If this is the case for you, when in your working week is the mismatch most apparent? Which of your needs, talents, and interests feel most thwarted in your current role?

Change can be so difficult that it's tempting to either skip the important steps, or to procrastinate. To manage these temptations, a project plan can be both organizing and motivating. The project plan could consist of a simple table similar to Table 9.1.

Table 9.1 Project plan

Stage	How?	By when?
Revisit self-knowledge		
Re-explore & longlist the options		
Shortlist & investigate the options		
Make the decision		
Implement the decision		

Self-knowledge revisited

We believe that the bigger a decision is, the more important it is that it is based on robust self-knowledge. Re-visiting the self-knowledge stage doesn't mean starting again but involves asking, 'Who am I *now*?' 'What do I *now* know about myself that I may not have known before?' Now is a good opportunity to consider what you don't enjoy or find fulfilling, what makes you feel anxious, frustrated, or doesn't interest you sufficiently. Alongside, you also need to ask yourself what *do* you enjoy or find stimulating? The self-knowledge exercises described in Chapter 2 can now be adapted.

The lifeline exercise

If you have already drawn a career lifeline, you can add a section to represent your recent life and work, annotating it with any new insights or perspectives.

The writing exercise

Writing remains a versatile way to reveal your implicit self-knowledge. Some additional topics you may want to include:

- New insights about yourself—what you now know you need from work
- activities, responsibilities, work relationships, or topics you want more of—or less of
- In their book, *A Job to* Love,[16] School of Life suggest that as children, we have more free time and censor our choices less than adults. So recalling the choices you made as a child can provide you with information that could be useful. What sort of play or activity did you enjoy if you had some free time away from electronic devices? What does this tell you about the sorts of activity you're naturally drawn to?

The achievements exercise

The achievements exercise, being shorter than the writing exercise, is sometimes preferred by doctors. It involves describing the small things that mattered most to you or made you feel proud, detailing your own role, your skills and talents that made the difference. It's okay if other people wouldn't consider your achievements important. You may recall Caroline's example of feeling proud of her role in helping a particular doctor, who experienced mental health problems, find a rewarding career beyond clinical medicine.

The experience log

Busy doctors with little time for writing can usually manage to log their experiences. It can be helpful to include non-work episodes and to cover a range of experiences—including those that make you feel stressed.

Holland's vocational interests

The tool we now want to describe straddles two of our stages—self-knowledge and exploration. We earlier argued that personality is a poor indicator of which medical specialties might suit which person. But 'person-environment fit' is an important concept in career research and was the area of interest of psychologist John Holland. For decades from the 1950s onwards, Holland investigated the types of work activities people found rewarding, identifying six dimensions that have been replicated in subsequent studies. The dimensions are not personality traits but are vocational interests. They have come to be known by the acronym, RIASEC.[17]

- **R**ealistic individuals are interested in working with things rather than with abstract ideas or people. They're typically active individuals both at work and in leisure.

- **Investigative** people are analytical, intellectual, mathematical, or scientific. They tend to want to solve complex or abstract problems at work and in leisure.
- **Artistic** people generally want to work intuitively using their aesthetic competencies in various forms—written, visual, musical, built environment, dance, etc.
- **Social** types prefer to work with people and generally enjoy helping others, drawing upon their communication skills.
- **Enterprising** people enjoy leading others. They tend to be interested in people's opinions, sales, marketing, and persuasion.
- **Conventional** people are interested in the conventions associated with how information is presented and handled. They are often skilful in handling data.

As well as people, job roles can be given RIASEC codes to signify the RIASEC type of people who typically occupy the roles. The Self-Directed Search (listed at the end of the chapter) is one of the many online inventories that use Holland's RIASEC classification. Individuals are coded according to their top three vocational interests generating a list of vocations attracting people with that code.

We have noticed that doctors can feel frustrated when they are presented with a list of occupations that includes medical roles. This is highly likely to happen and may suggest the doctors had come into medicine for logical reasons. Overall, it makes sense to see vocational interest questionnaires as one of a number of tools—which don't tell you 'the answer' but can instead generate useful ideas to explore.

Pulling the information together

Once you have updated your self-knowledge, it is helpful to summarize the key information on one sheet. You will recall from Chapter 2 that this is a process similar to that of selection panels when they write person specifications—but here it is *you* who is stating your personal criteria for judging *job roles*. You may find it helpful to use one of the tables (Table 2.4 or 2.5) in Chapter 2 which can be downloaded by searching for this book's ISBN 9780198884873 at https://academic.oup.com (see 'Additional Online Content' for further information).

Conversations with significant others

We earlier suggested that the self-knowledge exercises are best done on your own. But where there is also a process of identity change to be navigated, being supported is likely to be extremely important. It can be hard to predict how supportive different people will be, but you will have a sense of the key people you need to talk to. If a person may themselves be affected by your career decision, the conversation may feel like the beginning of an important negotiation. A spouse may need to alter their own career plan, work pattern, or geographic location to accommodate the changes you are contemplating. We suggest that you:

- Talk about the dilemma, its impact on you, and any emotional effects.
- Talk about what you need, your goals for work.
- Talk about how the person could support you
- Listen to what they have to say even if you don't agree with it and discuss how a compromise, if needed, could be made.

Box 9.2 **From bedside to bench**

Angus is a non-clinical immunologist who considers, with hindsight, that he originally chose to study medicine to please his parents. He didn't enjoy his preclinical course but reasoned it might be a means to an end. With an incisive and enquiring mind, he eventually found intellectual stimulation during his BSc year. This told him that he needed to find his way into research—but how to go about it? At the time the MB PhD (a programme allowing students to take an academic path) did not exist. Career advice for medical students also seemed not to have yet been invented. A tutor suggested becoming a physician before embarking on a clinical research career—a suggestion which made change sound almost impossible.

Alarm bells rang as the clinical course progressed. Students seemed to be discouraged from questioning how things were done. It was obligatory to underplay any feelings of discomfort so Angus ignored the warning signals, thinking of them as challenges to be survived.

Angus found his F1-equivalent stressful. As the year progressed he felt a million miles from his peers who enjoyed delivering patient care while he did not. He again sought advice, this time from his histopathology professor. His advice was to train in histopathology as a route to becoming an academic. Angus leapt at the opportunity and once training in the specialty, began to feel comfortable with the path. The nature of the tasks in histopathology suited him well. Angus relaxed into working better hours with colleagues who had questioning minds and talked openly about the limits of medical knowledge.

The journey took a further turn. The histopathology department subscribed to *Nature* and one month, the headline article claimed to solve a scientific question that interested Angus: antigen presentation. At the same moment, a colleague applied for PhD funding. Angus did the same. By chance, a cutting-edge immunology lecture was delivered by a guest speaker, allowing the final piece of the puzzle to click into place. Within a week of visiting the speaker's lab, Angus had applied for funding to study for a PhD with him, kick-starting his own academic career.

The case study in Box 9.2 suggests change can be a long process.

In Angus' case, the destination was clear but the route circuitous. But what if you don't yet know what directions are even possible?

Exploration

Exploration can now require considerable ingenuity. In contrast to the medical specialties which are neatly presented online, the information about other types of job role is much more widely distributed. For inspiration and ideas, you'll need to carry out numerous online searches, read books and articles, talk to people, or listen to TED talks and podcasts. It's helpful to be organized, keeping notes, and bookmarking websites.

Time limited or forever?

Are you considering a trial period or you are looking to make a forever decision? For some, it's helpful to keep open the option of a return to clinical medicine. If so, your Training Programme Director or Head of School could be consulted about the possibility of a period 'Out of Programme' so as to retain your training number. An Out of Programme for Career Break (OOPC) is—at least in theory— 'a break for a designated and agreed period to pursue other interests e.g. domestic responsibilities, industry etc.'[18]

Less usual medical specialties

In our work with doctors, we have found that even when doctors need to make a change, they sometimes find that other job roles don't compare favourably with medical roles. In spite of the stresses and strains, doctors often experience a deep sense of meaning through their work.[19] Such a realization can be a reason to re-explore the full range of medical specialties rather than assuming that your earlier doubts necessitate giving up medicine entirely.

Checking the competition ratios may show some specialties to be highly competitive. If so, it is worth studying the selection criteria and a considering how to strengthen your application. Other specialties may appear insufficiently competitive. If this feels like a problem, it's worth asking yourself if competition needs to be this important to you. For whose sake must you prove yourself? How long-lasting might be the advantages of winning a competition? Could you contemplate applying to a less competitive specialty, perhaps setting the bar high in a different way?

Non-traditional medical roles or beyond

To explore roles for doctors outside those in the NHS, look to organizations like Medic Footprints, listed at the end of the chapter. This organization specializes in providing information about diverse work roles including those in the pharmaceutical sector, consultancy work, medicolegal work, and entrepreneurship, among others.

Directories of job roles

We suggest several websites at the end of the chapter which list the range of jobs and careers that exist, sometimes broken down by sector. Visiting them can prompt you to think more broadly. This is valuable as the full range of job roles has often become invisible to doctors, immersed as they are, in the medical world.

Previously considered roles

Think about all the job roles you have ever considered, including those you contemplated before applying to study medicine. What attracted you to these different roles and what put you off? Might you have rejected these alternatives because of assumptions about where they might lead? Even if you don't plan to revisit those particular roles, wondering why you had once considered them may help clarify something about your interests.

Studying

After years training and studying, it's uncommon in our experience for doctors to want to study further. And with student loans to pay off, a period of further study may be unaffordable (Figure 9.2). Occasionally the inspiration does arise—or is necessary to gain access to a field. Medic Footprints cautions against undertaking study for its own sake.[20] Having to upload evidence of skills and courses for years, doctors may come to over-value qualifications. It's worth wondering if you can reach a goal without further training. Could you learn on the job or undertake training later on?

The exploration stage may be slower and more iterative than it is when it concerns only the medical specialties. As you explore, try to create a longlist of roles that attract you. To these, you can apply your personal criteria for job roles, adding those that appear to fulfil your criteria to your shortlist. Typically it's helpful to have more than one option to investigate.

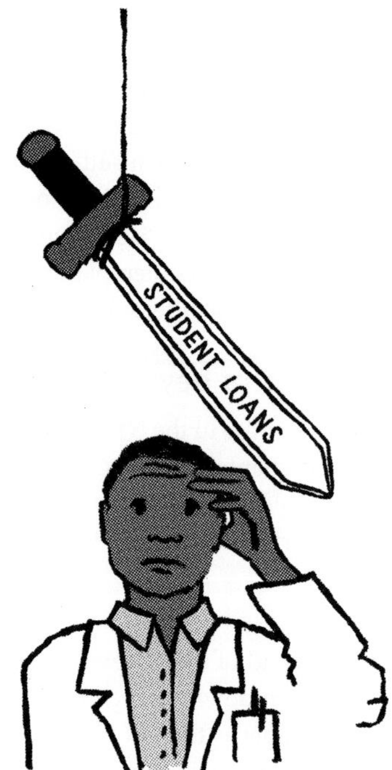

Figure 9.2 Can I afford to study?

Investigation

Outside the world of medicine, the investigation stage perhaps has a less collegiate feel, and informational interviews can be trickier to set up. The contact details for individuals rarely appear on websites and you may receive few replies from generic email addresses. It can be helpful to reach out to friends of friends or of relatives.

Presuming you do manage to find somebody to talk to about a job role that's of interest to you, draw up some questions you'd like to ask them. Keep in mind that they will be curious about you, perhaps wondering why you're considering 'giving it all up'. Even if you feel burnt out, try to give a balanced account of the journey, touching on the wealth of experience you have to offer. Some general questions (to which you can add your own) might be—

- What does a typical good and bad day look like?
- Where could a role like this lead?
- What gives people in these roles job satisfaction?
- What are the challenges and frustrations?
- How do you measure success?
- What preoccupies the seniors?
- How has the role changed? How might it change in future?
- Could you tell me something about your own career journey …

Decision-making

In Part 1 we discussed 'decision hygiene'. There are strong arguments for applying decision hygiene techniques now. You'll recall that once the relevant data is in, intuition can be given free rein. If intuition evades you, you can put in some structure, using an options appraisal or imagining various different futures (see Chapter 5).

Implementing your decision

The curriculum vitae

- In the medical world, CVs were long ago replaced by portal-based applications. Doctors creating CVs tend to worry about the veracity of the content, giving too little attention to the layout. In the non-medical world, it's important to sell yourself—so language and layout are important. Fortunately, hints and professional help for CV writing are easy to find online.

- Create a new version of your CV for each post. This doesn't mean re-writing it from scratch every time but fine-tuning it so that your suitability for the job in question jumps out of the page.

- Give a positive account of your medical career and the reasons for your change in direction. A future employer wants to feel that you are drawn to the new job rather than desperate to stop working as a doctor.

Try to emphasize the skills you think will be helpful for the job role. If you have written a paper or participated in a quality improvement project or even organized an on-call rota, consider the skills you drew upon with these tasks. You may have researched and summarized existing knowledge, analysed data, presented findings to expert audiences. To deliver clinical care you will have solved complex problems, worked quickly, most likely as part of a team in a rapidly changing environment.

Selection

Given the competition to train to become a doctor, it can be surprising to find competition for non-medical roles too. The selection process is often lengthier than for medical roles, involving multiple interviews sometimes at an assessment centre. You may be asked to take a cognitive ability test (CAT) or to complete a personality questionnaire. Assessment centres commonly invite applicants to participate in exercises with each other, developing ideas in a group in which no leader has been assigned. It's possible to guess the criteria that will be used to judge individuals which may include listening, understanding, and expressing ideas– qualities many doctors have.

Interviews often follow a situational format, 'Tell us about a time when you handled [a certain type of situation].' Reading the job description and person specification may allow you to speculate about what could be asked. You might prepare by writing down some possible responses, speaking your ideas aloud, or you could persuade someone to carry out a practice interview with you. Plan what you would like to ask at the interview.

Job offers

If a post is offered to you, carefully consider if you want to take it up or if you first have questions to ask. You may have the chance to negotiate some of the practicalities of the post—your hours, your work base, training, or pay.

Culture shock

Change, even when welcome, can be difficult—so much so that we sometimes speak of 'culture shock'. Anthropologist Kalervo Oberg, who originated the concept in his studies of people moving geographically, noticed an initial positive honeymoon period followed by periods of crisis and recovery. Defined as 'a sudden, unexpected and surprising set of mainly negative emotions and cognitions associated with encountering a new environment',[21] culture shock applies equally to change in relation to work. A study of PhD students moving out of academia found around half to experience culture shock.[22] The issues the employees struggled with included loss of autonomy, approaches to presenting evidence, teamworking, and organizational values and hierarchies.

It makes sense to be prepared to experience culture shock. Consider:

♦ whether a honeymoon stage—a period of confusion or frustration seems to be happening.

♦ asking colleagues about some of the unspoken cultural expectations of the team or organization.

- that building up your professional network is likely to be helpful.
- taking up mentoring if it is available.
- that coming from medicine is an opportunity to ask questions with genuine curiosity.
- that it may feel strange not to be an expert in a new field. It may help if you can develop a growth mindset (discussed in Chapter 8).

One possible barrier: procrastination

We have previously considered how cognitive shortcuts can interfere with decision-making. Continuity Bias, sometimes known as the Sunk Cost Fallacy, is one such shortcut. It is our tendency to resist giving up something for which we worked hard—even if in doing so the reward promises to be greater. One temptation, then, is to procrastinate, leading to more uncertainty. At worst, we might even end up running out of time. In order to tackle this:

- Make a project plan that includes time frames for the different stages.
- Try one or two thought experiments:
  - Imagine you did not make the change under consideration. Instead you continued to experience misgivings or career regret for the rest of your career. What might this be like? How would you cope and adapt? Is this something you feel able to manage? What are the alternatives? If you were to pursue an alternative, how might things work out?
  - Imagine what you might have done had you not trained as a doctor. What might your life have been like at the various stages? How might things be now? What might life be like in future?

Summary

Not all doctors who consider leaving will do so. We know from following up previous clients that although moving on is the right decision for some doctors it can also pose significant challenges. Exploring non-medical options often takes longer as the options are not set out as neatly as the medical specialties.

By imposing a structure and method on the messiness, it *is* possible to find a way forward that is right for you. Some doctors feel guilty about moving on as they have a tremendous sense of duty to continue in the NHS. Certainly the health service would collapse if *every*body who felt frustrated or who experienced burnout left. But as this is unlikely to happen, choices remain for those who feel the need to explore alternative options to medicine.

References

1. **Surman, G., Goldacre, M.J., & Lambert, T.W.** (2017). UK-trained junior doctors' intentions to work in UK medicine: questionnaire surveys, three years after graduation. *J R Soc Med.* **110**(12):493–500. https://doi.org/10.1177/0141076817738500
2. **Lambert, T.W., Smith, F., & Goldacre, M.J.** (2018). Why doctors consider leaving UK medicine: qualitative analysis of comments from questionnaire surveys three years after graduation. *J R Soc Med.* **111**(1):18–30. DOI: 10.1177/0141076817738502

3. **British Medical Association** (2024). When a doctor leaves: tackling the cost of attrition. https://www.bma.org.uk/media/gsmfle1o/tackling-the-cost-of-attrition-uks-health-servi ces.pdf

4. **General Medical Council** (2021). Completing the picture report. https://www.gmc-uk.org/about/what-we-do-and-why/data-and-research/research-and-insight-archive/com pleting-the-picture-report

5. **Jewett, E.A., Brotherton, S.E., & Ruch-Ross, H.** (2011). A national survey of 'inactive' physicians in the United States of America: enticements to re-entry. *Hum Resour Health.* **9**:1–10. DOI:10.1186/1478-4491-9-7

6. **Pathmanathan, A., & Snelling, I.** (2023). Exploring reasons behind UK doctors leaving the medical profession: a series of qualitative interviews with former UK doctors. *BMJ Open.* **13**(9):e068202.

7. **Zeelenberg, M., & Pieters, R.** (2007). A theory of regret regulation 1.0. *J Consum Psychol.* **17**(1):3–18.

8. **Budjanovcanin, A., Rodrigues, R., & Guest, D.** (2019). A career with a heart: exploring occupational regret. *J Manag Psychol.* **34**(3).156–169. https://doi.org/10.1108/ JMP- 02-2018-0105

9. **Peirce, G.L., Desselle, S.P., … & Bolino, M.** (2012). Identifying psychological contract breaches to guide improvements in faculty recruitment, retention, and development. *Am J Pharm Educ.* **76**(6):108. https://doi.org/10.5688/ajpe766108

10. **Dyrbye, L.N., Burke, S.E., … & Van Ryn, M.** (2018). Association of clinical specialty with symptoms of burnout and career choice regret among US resident physicians. *JAMA.* **320**(11):1114–1130. DOI: doi:10.1001/jama.2018.12615

11. **Rousseau, D.M.** (1989). Psychological and implied contracts in organizations. *Empl Responsib Rights J.* **2**:121–139. DOI: 10.1007/BF01384942

12. **Rusbult, C.E., & Farrell, D.** (1983). A longitudinal test of the investment model: The impact on job satisfaction, job commitment, and turnover of variations in rewards, costs, alternatives, and investments. *J Appl Psychol.* **68**(3):429. https://doi.org/10.1037/ 0021-9010.68.3.429

13. **Kübler-Ross, E.** (1970) *On death and dying.* Tavistock Publications.

14. **Maciejewski, P.K., Zhang, B., … & Prigerson, H. G.** (2007). An empirical examination of the stage theory of grief. *JAMA.* **297**(7):716–723.DOI: 10.1001/jama.297.7.716

15. **Gerada, C.** (2022). Doctors' identity and barriers to seeking care when unwell. *Br J Psychiatry.* **220**(1):7–9. DOI:10.1192/bjp.2021.52

16. **School of Life** (2017). *A job to love.* School of Life.

17. **Nauta, M.M.** (2010). The development, evolution, and status of Holland's theory of vocational personalities: reflections and future directions for counseling psychology. *J Couns Psychol.* **57**(1):11. https://doi.org/10.1037/a0018213

18. **NHS England** (n.d.). Workforce, training and education. https://www.hee.nhs.uk/our-work/dentists-training/delivering-greater-flexibility/out-programme

19. **Horowitz, C.R., Suchman, A.L., … & Frankel, R.M.** (2003). What do doctors find meaningful about their work? *Ann Int Med.* **138**(9):772–775. DOI: 10.7326/ 0003-4819-138-9-200305060-00028

20. **Medic Footprints** (n.d.). Doctors leaving medicine: do you need more qualifications to start an alternative career? https://medicfootprints.org/podcasts/doctors-leaving-medic ine-qualifications-alternative-career/

21. **Furnham, A.** (2019). Culture shock: a review of the literature for practitioners. *Psychology.* **10**(13):1832–1855. https://doi.org/10.4236/psych.2019.1013119

22. **Skakni, I., Inouye, K., & McAlpine, L.** (2022). PhD holders entering non-academic workplaces: organisational culture shock. *Stud High Educ.* **47**(6):1271–1283. DOI: 10.1080/03075079.2021.1876650

Further information

Medic Footprints Alternative and diverse career opportunities for doctors https://medicfootprints.org

New Scientist careers https://jobs.newscientist.com/careers

O*Net Online (USA) https://www.onetonline.org

Prospects Graduate careers (UK) https://www.prospects.ac.uk/job-profiles

Self-Directed Search https://self-directed-search.com

UK Government: All Sectors https://jobhelp.campaign.gov.uk/improve-your-chances-of-getting-a-job/all-sectors/

Chapter 10

What if I've chosen the wrong specialty?

There is something I don't know
    that I am supposed to know.
I don't know *what* it is I don't know,
    and yet am supposed to know,
and I feel I look stupid
    if I seem both not to know it
        and not know *what* it is I don't know.
Therefore I pretend I know it.
    This is nerve-racking
    since I don't know what I must pretend to know.
Therefore I pretend to know everything.

R.D. Laing[1]

In the last chapter we considered the needs of the group of doctors who are considering leaving the profession. But there is another group whose needs we want to consider: those who select a specialty only to wonder if it is right for them. It makes most sense to consider a couple of common problems before moving on to consider whether it is actually necessary to change specialty. This chapter can be read together with Chapter 12, which tackles stress, mental health difficulties, well-being, and resilience.

We start with the pain of the sense many of us have that we don't know enough, sometimes known as imposter syndrome or imposter phenomenon. As we move on to consider personality, we concern ourselves less with your own personality than with those of the people around you and also the team's 'personality'. We recognize though, that for some doctors there is a sense of being mismatched—of being a square peg in a round hole. This can feel like a serious problem that needs addressing. But it is one which can benefit from the same structured approach we have used elsewhere in the book.

The pain of not knowing

Doctors are expected to hit the ground running. They must learn at lightning speed. And there's often a tension between asking questions, which can feel exposing versus relying on prior knowledge or 'first principles', which can mean learning less. This is an example of cognitive dissonance—the discomfort we experience when faced with important but contradictory ideas.[2] When experiencing cognitive dissonance, a common solution is to be consciously aware of one side of the equation, ignoring the other. So under pressure, we might convince ourselves that we must ask about and look up *everything*. Or we might do the opposite. Today's generation of doctors may be more adept at addressing *both* sides of the equation, 'I know this, but not that. I don't know this hospital's protocol; please tell me where I can find it'. Too often though, it's hard to find somebody to whom to address these questions. Another factor is that all this can be exhausting. If you search your own recollections of being new in a post (as Naomi did in Box 10.1), it's not only about factual knowledge, but also about how things are done—and even who's who.

Many of us are reluctant to ask for help. Yet help did materialize for Naomi (Box 10.1) in this instance. So *why* are we reluctant to ask for help? One reason may be

Box 10.1 **Naomi's start in psychiatry**

My sweaty hands gripped the edge of the desk on this inauspicious day, the day of my first psychiatric outpatient clinic. But what was this? A doorbell? By a strange coincidence, the clinic room door opened a crack and the receptionist appeared, wide eyed, 'Is everything alright?' It was *not a coincidence*: I'd pressed the emergency buzzer that nobody had thought to mention. I had foolishly summoned emergency help. But no matter—my patient was not feeling particularly patient, so we pressed on. She irritably rattled off all the pressures she faced, being the stage manager of Bolshoi Ballet, as they prepared to perform in the most dangerous war zone at the time. I sympathized. But it sounded odd. It took me far too long to realize how unwell my patient was—my first-ever patient I was seeing in clinic, outside the security of the ward. What should I do? The clinical team were nowhere to be seen. Only the receptionist was there, still jumpy after the false alarm.

The ward work wasn't going well either. My face-blindness (prosopagnosia, though undiagnosed) caused settling-in problems. With no name badges, who was a staff member and who was a patient? Everybody seemed as depressed as each other—including me! Reader, I cried—in the office of a gentle professor who politely asked, 'Are you keeping up with your reading?' What a daft question, I thought—hardly relevant! But perhaps that professor's question was intended to distract both of us from the embarrassment of my tears. In those days, it was unusual to cry at work. Perhaps my tears communicated something because as if by magic, my next placement was on a ward, legendary in the hospital, for its less frantic pace—where the staff wore name badges and were kind.

imposter syndrome—or we might more accurately refer to it as imposter phenomenon (as this is clearly not a medical condition). First described by psychotherapists, Pauline Clance and Suzanne Imes,[3] imposter syndrome/phenomenon has to do with fearing being 'found out' as lacking—being found not to possess the expertise you feel you are supposed to have.

Imposter phenomenon is associated with lacking confidence, anxiety and, for those who set themselves impossibly high standards, can lead to depression.[4] Originally described in a cohort of women, imposter feelings are not gender-specific. Those in any under-represented group may be more vulnerable[5] and we also know that the phenomenon occurs in doctors.[6] The case study in Box 10.2 is intended as an example.

Becoming aware that you are experiencing imposter phenomenon as Jasmine did can in itself be a great help. Naming the phenomenon brings an acceptance that you are *clearly* not an imposter. Once in the open, it is heartening to find that many peers have the same experience. It can be even more helpful if seniors are able to share with you their own experiences of imposter feelings.

> ### Box 10.2 **Apply only if you speak with 'Received Pronunciation'**
>
> Now with her Certificate of Completion of Training (CCT) in General Surgery, Jasmine was in her 'grace period'. It was time to tackle what felt like the last hurdle—applying for a consultant post. Jasmine planned to apply for a post at a local hospital she knew well. She'd worked there on and off for years and got on well with the staff. But a friend had mentioned a soon-to-be advertised opportunity: a maternity cover locum consultant post in a prestigious teaching hospital. Jasmine met all the essential criteria but the list of desirable criteria was so long, she couldn't possibly fulfil all of them. Bemoaning this fact in the pub, Jasmine's friends insisted she had a fair chance. One friend suggested Jasmine might be suffering from a touch of imposter syndrome. From a working-class background and the first in her family to go to university, Jasmine took the idea seriously. She was well aware of the class divide in medicine. Jasmine was occasionally mocked for her accent, once in front of an audience. She tried her best to speak 'properly' but at the same time sensed that patients appreciated her 'being one of us'. But what about the hiring committee? Might *they* see Jasmine as an outsider?
>
> Reading an article online, *Rising to the Level of Your* Incompetence,[6] Jasmine could see herself as one of the cases—vulnerable to imposter syndrome on account of her social class. Though an unwelcome thought, the insight did help Jasmine face up to the possibility that she might be holding herself back in a way that was potentially career-sabotaging. So, bracing herself, Jasmine chose the ambitious route. She was duly appointed—and later, to the next role: a substantive consultant post. Jasmine could imagine herself working happily at the local hospital. But she might have had a nagging sense that the choice had been made with too much credence given to the imposter syndrome and its anxiety.

If, after thinking about imposter syndrome, you still feel there could be a problem with your own ability, it may be helpful to ask for feedback, preferably from more than one person. When it comes to interpreting the feedback, keep in mind the Dunning–Kruger effect, discussed in Chapter 8, which suggests it's common for other people to rate your skill at a level lower than your own self-ratings. It may seem unlikely that you can both worry about not being good enough and at the same time rate your skills higher than other people's ratings. But there's every reason for both the imposter phenomenon and the Dunning–Kruger effect to occur in the same person. This would be an example of cognitive dissonance. At a practical level: don't be disheartened if others rate you lower than you rate yourself. The important issue is whether your skills are at the level expected for your stage.

Personalities and team culture

Every team or work context is unique. For one thing, each is made up of a particular combination of people with their distinct personalities. By personality, we mean the relatively stable ways in which people differ from each other. To add to the complexity, the situations we find ourselves in also explain our behaviour to some extent.[7] A person may surprise us by behaving quite differently in different contexts. A senior doctor might seem argumentative or tetchy in a particular meeting, then in a 1:1 situation, they might be kind and friendly. That may be all well and good, but how often do the less pressured 1:1 moments occur in practice?

There is also the team culture to consider. Culture is the 'set of shared beliefs, values, and attitudes that shape and are shaped by individual and collective actions within organizations'. The shared beliefs, values, and attitudes, socially constructed as they may be, come to be seen as 'reality'.[8] A team culture can be so distinctive that we might think of the team as having a personality of its own. If you encounter a problem with a team, it's worth considering whether it has to do with the rules and practices of the team, or whether it mostly crops up with a particular person—both are possible.

Whether you encounter a problem with a person or a team, it's tempting to make yourself small and quiet (especially if shame, one of the more difficult emotions, sets in). Alternatively, you could ask yourself:

- When, in what situations, and with whom does this problem occur?
- Within this particular team, who does what?
- How does my role interact with other people's roles?
- Is there anything about my approach or style of communication I could alter?
- Do colleagues experience similar difficulties?
- Who has the position and authority to help?
- What steps can I take?

When work and life converge

Our lives outside work go on irrespective of whether or not we have just started in a new post and feel overwhelmed. At certain life stages many events happen at around the same time. Some may be very positive events—getting married or having a child—but even positive life events require adaptation. It's helpful to consider the following:

- How would somebody in a different kind of job cope?

- How would a role model cope? (Recall a role model is someone you aspire to be like)

- Who can you talk to?

- Ideas circulate in our cultures about what we must do—some helpful, some are unhelpful, but quite insistent. Can you identify any unhelpful ideas that people have suggested (such as—for example—the notion that a pre-school child must only be cared for by their mother). What can you do to minimize the impact of others' unhelpful comments?

What if the specialty I chose *really* doesn't seem right?

What, if upon considering the various possibilities, you are left thinking the specialty you've chosen isn't right for you? If so, it's helpful to face up to that possibility and list what issues you find uncomfortable. For balance, you could also list what you find interesting or rewarding.

If you feel overwhelmed by the scale of the change you are thinking about, consider if a *small* change could make a significant difference? A smaller change may be less disruptive than a larger change. Such a change could be a change of location, a change of team, or of focus. For some, a small change will not suffice—a bigger, or even a radical change is needed. It is worth considering:

- When do you expect to rotate? Could you sample—through shadowing—the next (or a subsequent) leg of your journey?

- Is there a person or team in your specialty whose style is fresh and interesting? What could you learn from this person about how to approach your work, or about future career directions in your specialty?

- If you had the time to read widely or attend conferences, might you find an area in your specialty that truly interested you?

- What is the range of sub-specialties open to you?

- Would you enjoy taking on significant management or educational responsibilities in your trust so that your clinical duties will come to occupy a smaller part of your overall job plan?

- Do you have the potential to be an academic? Would you find your specialty more conducive as a research clinician? If so, how could you find out about this option?

- Could you use your specialty experience in a role outside of the NHS, e.g. in the pharmaceutical sector?

- Are you thinking about changing specialty? Do your training and qualifications allow you to enter a new specialty at a point other than the very beginning?

- Is there any merit in starting afresh in an entirely new specialty? Our experience working with doctors is that it is easier to change specialty at an earlier stage in the training. If you feel you are at risk of procrastinating, you may want to return to the thought experiments discussed in Chapter 9.

Having previously investigated the options, you may inwardly sigh at the thought of further informational interviews. It can be hard to decide who to talk to. Many who seek a significant change feel concerned about privacy. But consider that there are people who have a duty of care for you. You could ask for an assurance of confidentiality. Conversations at this point may feel quite different: with the benefit of experience, your questions will be more nuanced and you will be better able to interpret what you hear.

Summary

We have used this chapter to outline some of the issues that can interfere with your progress in, and enjoyment of, the specialty you've chosen. Many doctors make good progress towards their goals and don't question their commitment at all. If you do find yourself unsure about your chosen specialty, it is first wise to look at a number of possible causes of your discomfort before concluding that you are on the wrong path. Could you be experiencing imposter feelings? Does your discomfort have to do with any particular colleague or team? Is life throwing you curve balls outside work? Or perhaps it really is the case that you have selected a specialty that turned out to be a poor match for your individual needs.

As our careers can span almost a whole lifetime, it makes perfect sense to take steps to ensure that your specialty (or sub-specialty) choice is one in which you can thrive and grow, rather than a line of work which, at best, you must endure.

References

1. **Laing, R.D.** (1971). *Knots*. Penguin Books.
2. **Festinger, L.** (1957). *A theory of cognitive dissonance*. Row and Peterson.
3. **Clance, P.R., & Imes, S.A.** (1978). The imposter phenomenon in high achieving women: dynamics and therapeutic intervention. *Psychol Psychother Theory Res Pract.* **15**(3):241. https://doi.org/10.1037/h0086006
4. **Neureiter, M., & Traut-Mattausch, E.** (2016). An inner barrier to career development: preconditions of the impostor phenomenon and consequences for career development. *Front Psychol.* 2016;7:173631. DOI: 10.3389/fpsyg.2016.00048
5. **Mullangi, S., & Jagsi, R.** (2019). Imposter syndrome: treat the cause, not the symptom. *JAMA.***322**(5):403–404. 10.1001/jama.2019.9788
6. **LaDonna, K.A., Ginsburg, S., & Watling, C.** (2018). 'Rising to the level of your incompetence': what physicians' self-assessment of their performance reveals about the imposter syndrome in medicine. *Acad Med.* **93**(5):763–768. DOI: 10.1097/ACM.0000000000002046
7. **Wagerman, S.A., & Funder, D.C.** (2009). Personality psychology of situations. In: Corr, P.J. & Matthews, G., eds. *The Cambridge handbook of personality psychology*. Cambridge University Press; 27–42. https://doi.org/10.1017/CBO9780511596544.005
8. **Alvesson, M.** (2012). *Understanding organizational culture*. Sage Publications.

Chapter 11

UK doctors working overseas

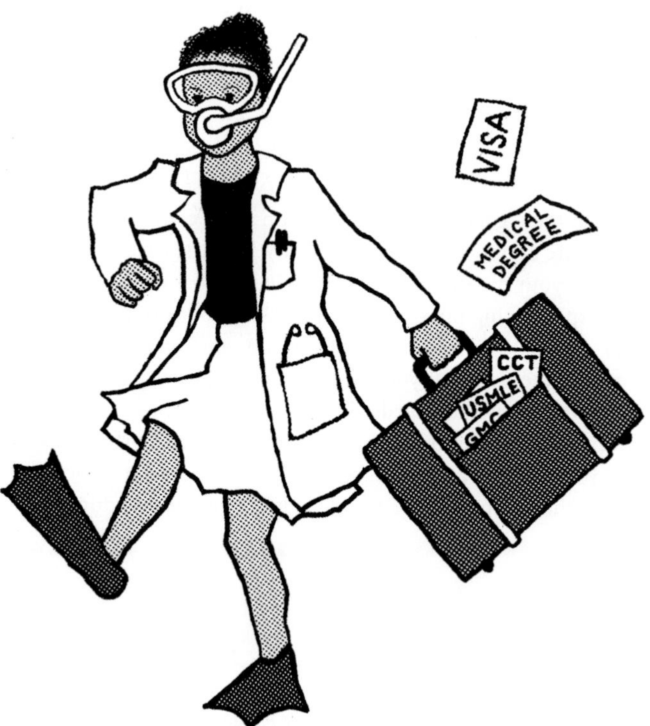

Figure 11.1 Travel can mean choosing your own baggage.

The world needs doctors! And the doctoring role, being strikingly similar from country to country, can make medical qualifications potentially exportable (Figure 11.1). In this chapter we consider how many doctors make use of their medical qualification to practice in other countries. We ask *why* doctors want to travel and whether travelling lives up to their hopes. The internet is awash with tips and tricks—some of which we summarize here. We take the view that career planning doesn't need to stop if you're in another country—even if that country is in a different hemisphere. There'll naturally be times when you'll be taking in the landscape and properly immersing yourself in the new culture. But you will also want to capture and make best use of the professional experience that you're accumulating to further your career in that country, or to pack it up and bring it back with you to the UK.

Who travels?

A 2021 paper reported that around 4% of doctors leave the UK medical workforce each year.[1] Half leave to work outside the UK. A survey done several generations ago suggests that travelling is not a new trend. In 1970, doctors travelled for similar reasons: the love of travelling, a better lifestyle, better pay, and better opportunities. Almost a fifth of the doctors surveyed felt dissatisfied with the NHS.[2] We see, then, that the experience of previous generations chimes uncannily with that of today's doctors. One difference, however, is that there has been a reduction in the proportion of doctors progressing straight from their foundation training into a training in one of the specialties. The number of doctors taking what is now called the 'F3 year' rose from 17% in 2010 to 65% in 2019.[3] And for many of doctors, the 'F3 year' is the perfect moment to travel.

Medical workforce planners must feel the need to keep a watchful eye on the numbers as one of their tasks is to encourage UK graduates back to the UK. A GMC-commissioned study found a third of F3 doctors take up posts outside the UK. There is no particular gender difference between the groups. Travelling doctors who are non-UK graduates are slightly older, in their 30s, and more likely to leave the UK permanently, returning to their home countries.[3] UK graduates are more likely to travel while in their 20s, their destinations most commonly being English-speaking Australia and New Zealand.

Do doctors fulfil their dreams by travelling?

Surveys also tell us what travelling doctors are looking for. Many doctors report envisioning the next stage of their training as an intense period so for them the F3 year is a chance to take a break from training. Working abroad is an attractive way to step off the training-treadmill. Many see travel as providing an opportunity for personal growth alongside an opportunity to enhance professional skills.[3] The same is true for international medical graduates travelling to the UK whose hopes are similar.[1] The wish to broaden one's work experience and to find better working conditions appears universal.

What then, do UK doctors find when they travel abroad? Wilson et al. asked two hundred doctors this question.[4] Theirs was an unusual sample made up of doctors who had left a NHS training programme and who had ultimately trained in a specialty in Australia, New Zealand, Canada, or the US. More than half had previously experienced symptoms of burn-out. Most had gone on to recover in their adopted country and had come to feel valued and satisfied with their work-life balance. These findings echo those of an older study carried out by the UK Medical Careers Research Group who surveyed 38,821 UK doctors graduating between 1974 and 2005.[5] The researchers sent surveys to those doctors within the overall cohort who were registered to practise in New Zealand: a smaller sample of 419 doctors—of which 282 doctors responded to the survey. Forty-eight per cent of those responding had originally intended their stay in New Zealand to be temporary—but at the point of the survey, 89% expected to remain permanently. When the study was published in 2012 the headlines in the medical and mainstream presses de-cried the medical brain drain. But to put the figure in context, those expecting to permanently remain in New Zealand represented less than 1% of the overall cohort of doctors from which the smaller sample was drawn.

In a further study of over four thousand UK trained doctors taking a post-foundation training break (PFTB), 33% of those working clinically did so outside the UK for all or part of the year. The proportion doing so reduced to 23% as travel restrictions set in during the pandemic period.[6] In the group of doctors taking a PFTB, 60% saw themselves as stronger applicants on account of their travels. The recruiters also considered that doctors taking post-foundation training breaks tended to strengthen their applications, often being better able than competitors to demonstrate the required skills. So a period off the treadmill, whether or not you work abroad can be helpful. For the NHS however, there is a risk that the experience of travelling is so positive that doctors do not want to return.

Preparing to travel

So what are the practical steps worth taking prior to travelling? You may already know where you plan to go or you may feel inspired by other doctors' experience. Whatever your source of inspiration, your chance of getting work is greater in a country which needs additional doctors. You will naturally want to find out how the health service works in the countries under consideration. Not only will the service differ, but so will the structure of the training—including the names and duration of the training stages. The principle of competition will apply: a post in a smaller, rural hospital could be easier to be appointed to than a highly sought-after teaching-hospital post in a major city. Applying at the level of your competence and experience is also important.

When you speak to those who have already gone down your intended path, you'll be keen to discuss the beginning of the trip. It's worth also asking about their experience of returning to the UK as this is a transition that can be hard to navigate.

The paperwork

Paperwork often takes longer than expected. The British Medical Association (BMA) sensibly suggests written offers should be signed by both parties before travelling.[7] Though the BMA website offers some general guidance on contracts, their offer does not include checking contracts in non-UK jurisdictions. One potential hazard they point out is of being asked to undertake activities that could contravene international human rights or ethical standards. Members can email the BMA ethics department who may be able to comment on any proposed duties that raise concerns of this kind.[8] Questions about the visa requirements of the country you're considering should be addressed to the country's high commissioner or embassy.

Registration

In order to work as a doctor in another country, UK medical graduates need to request a Certificate of Good Standing from the GMC.[9] With regard to your UK registration and licence to practice, there appear to be choices between maintaining both of these, giving up just your licence to practice or giving up both.[10] Our anecdotal impression is that many doctors retain both their UK registration and licence to practise if they think it possible they will want to return to UK practice. It is worth talking to the GMC to ensure you understand the consequences of each choice.

To find the relevant information about a host country's registration process, try using the name of the country as a search term together with 'Medical Council', 'Medical Registrar', or 'Medical Association'.

Tasks that could be forgotten

Other tasks include: arranging medical indemnity; health and travel insurance; and immunizations. Communicating with HMRC may reduce the risk of overpaying or underpaying UK tax. The Student Loans Company will want to know your plans to determine your ongoing repayments. Seek advice from NHS Pensions if you hope to pay into your NHS pension while away.

What about agencies?

Travellers report finding medical recruitment agencies helpful. Some but not all may be able to help with registration, visas, paperwork, or even accommodation. However there's nothing to stop you contacting hospital human resources (HR) departments directly.

Working for a charity or NGO

You may be interested in working voluntarily for a charity or non-governmental organization in a lower income country. Doing so can give you a broader perspective and allow you to contribute to those whose lives are affected by poverty, food shortages, or other adversities. For the local healthcare system to benefit from visiting doctors, organizations often require a couple of years' post-foundation experience and a commitment of one to two years. Some organizations need doctors with specific clinical skills or specialty experience. A qualification in Tropical Medicine is often considered helpful. Choose an organization experienced enough to advise you on the practicalities and able to ensure that your visiting does not interfere with the local health service.

Schemes with links to the NHS

The NHS has a Global Engagement Partnership in England and similar departments in Wales and Scotland to support NHS staff who want to volunteer or undertake Global Health Fellowships in a lower income country (see Box 11.1 for a case study). We list these at the end of the chapter.

Box 11.1 The how and the where are for you to decide

Emmanuel is a UK trained British doctor of Nigerian heritage. Eager to work in Africa to broaden his experience, Emmanuel planned to get some training under his belt *before* travelling. With two years of ACCS (Acute Care Common Stem) training already completed and permission to take an out-of-programme experience, Emmanuel applied to become a Global Health Fellowship Volunteer. He considered undertaking a diploma in Tropical Medicine prior to travelling but the cost of doing so was prohibitive. Volunteering is an unpaid role with some paid-for perks, but there were many expenses that Emmanuel needed to meet himself. Emmanuel did, however, study in preparation for the trip, finding several inexpensive short courses covering the common endemic diseases, TB and HIV.

Emmanuel was matched with a placement at a rural hospital in Sierra Leone. He used the HEE toolkit to guide him through some of the logistics. What was most helpful was making contact with doctors who had previously volunteered, including one who had worked at the same hospital.

Some experience of culture shock was unavoidable because everything worked so very differently. But Emmanuel found the team highly skilled and welcoming. The pace of work was intense—more so than one could imagine. Emmanuel had exposure to diseases he had previously only seen in textbooks. There were moments in which Emmanuel experienced imposter syndrome (discussed in Chapter 10)—the feeling of knowing so little that you 'must' be an imposter. These feelings were triggered when Emmanuel's opinion was sought by his colleagues. This kind of situation unnerved him until he realized it was the team's way of making him feel welcome. Emmanuel found the supervision excellent. Although his supervisor was spread thinly over a large area so was not always available, Emmanuel could always ask for the advice from other members of the team.

Emmanuel was able to travel with colleagues to outreach clinics in isolated locations. Patients could be very sick and he was struck by the speed of many patients' recovery once they received the correct treatment. Patients and their families were often hugely resilient and inspiring.

Following his four-month attachment, Emmanuel travelled to Nigeria to meet his extended family, some of whom he had never before met. This was his first visit to his relatives since qualifying as a doctor. The trip kindled the itch for further travel and raised some interesting new career dilemmas.

F1 and F2 abroad

What if you want to spend one or both foundation years abroad? Your medical school will need to approve an F1 post planned to be abroad. You may be considering following the F1 with a standalone F2 post in the UK—in which case, talk to your foundation school about the availability of standalone F2 posts—which may vary from one year to the next.[11] F2 posts abroad require local (UK) foundation school permission if your intention is to return to UK training.

Both F1 and F2 posts entail finding an educational supervisor knowledgeable about the UK foundation training and willing to take on the responsibility. The e-portfolio then needs to be completed in the same way as you would in the UK. A helpful first-hand account written by a doctor who worked as an F2 doctor in Australia was available on the NHS Health Careers website[12] at the time of writing.

One approach to readying yourself for specialty training is to complete a Certificate of Readiness to Enter Specialty Training (CREST) form.[13] Doing so requires a high degree of organization as the rules surrounding the form and how it must be completed are exacting.

Travelling while already on a specialty training programme

Doctors like Emmanuel in our case study, who have already begun a UK core or specialty training, may want to travel. Those intending to return to their training must retain their training number. Doing so means negotiating a period 'out of programme' (OOP). The rules are specific,[14,15] so it's important to talk the issues through with the Training Programme Director or Head of School. Could your time out count towards your clinical training (OOPT)? Even if you are granted a period out of programme for clinical experience (OOPE), which does not count towards your training, the experience is still likely to broaden your knowledge and strengthen your future job applications. Options also exist to take time out for research (OOPR) or for a career break (OOPC). Whichever OOP is agreed, it is essential to be clear about the return-by date.

While travelling

Try to attend an induction where you can meet new colleagues and learn about how things work in the service. The colleagues you'll meet will be able to give invaluable informal tips including travel tips. There will be a lot to learn given how different the hospital and health service will be from that which you're used to. Even small details such as the drug names, the equipment, procedures or algorithms (or the lack of them) may differ. Keep a record of your skill development. It could be helpful if a senior could record the skills they've seen you competently perform—perhaps in their reference. Try to stay in touch with the seniors back home as well as with peers.

Career planning on the go

While travelling you may be inspired by various different career ideas. Some may be ideas you've previously considered, others may be completely new. It might seem like the career exercises we outlined in Chapter 2 belong to a different universe from the one you're in while you are travelling. So we suggest using just a couple. Keeping a private work-related journal and carrying out an experience log (at one time or another) are our more traveller-friendly exercises.

You'll recall that the exploration phase is about exploring the options available. The options in the country you're in will differ from those in the UK. As you embark on the exploration stage, make sure you tap into the information that's relevant to the country in which you plan to be for the next stage of your training.

Preparing to return

It has never before been easier to keep in touch with people and there are some real advantages to staying in touch with the medical friends you left behind in the UK. Finding out their plans can motivate you to visit the relevant UK websites keeping you abreast of the options and application windows. Travelling doctors tell us it can feel difficult to be motivated when abroad to spend time researching the UK system. There's a chance you'll fall into the trap of making a decision based only on the limited information you already have. Being in touch with friends may make this less likely. If you intend to return to training in the UK:

- Resist the temptation of gaining so much experience in a specialty that you become ineligible to train. Some specialties stipulate that doctors must have less than a certain amount of experience before entering CT1 or ST1 training. For this reason, it's important to check the person specifications on the official Health Education England (HEE) websites.

- A further reason for checking the person specifications is that specialties experiencing particular shortages of applicants sometimes introduce new ways to demonstrate the required competencies.

- Many of the official websites have a channel for asking questions.

- If you trained in another country in a specialty or in general practice and want to practice in the UK, you may be able to follow the portfolio route (CESR and CEGPR), discussed in Chapter 7.

What if I want to stay?

Like Joe, the case-study doctor in Box 11.2, some doctors decide to remain in their host country. Doing so can be a hard decision to make as there is the need to consider family and friends back home—although technology certainly makes it easier to be in touch.

Possible barriers to enhancing your career through travel

We have perhaps painted a picture—based upon the testimony of so many doctors—that it's good to travel. But what are the barriers?

Barrier No. 1: Other people's opinions

It seems too obvious to state that some people (perhaps most) are likely to be encouraging while others may discourage taking time off to travel. They may caution you about the risks to your career which can be tricky if those who discourage you are the people whose opinions matter the most.

- When you listen to other people's advice, especially if they take a discouraging position, it's worth wondering why they think what they do. Perhaps they are risk-averse or themselves dislike travel? Or perhaps they see training as a race. Maybe they are not aware of the opportunities in the country you're considering.

- Talk to a range of people including those who have themselves worked as doctors in other countries.

- Are the people you talk to giving you advice based on the outdated assumption that once you've completed foundation you should immediately progress to specialty training?

Barrier No. 2: Losing touch with home

Doctors have sometimes told us how hard it is to make specialty choices when working abroad. The same specialty can differ in different countries. Occasionally, technical issues such as poor internet connectivity can hamper your research. More often it's simply difficult to imagine the trip coming to an end. For those who have had difficult past experiences, it may be harder to disengage from the present to think about the future.[16] It may help to:

- Keep in touch with friends and colleagues
- Find a coach or mentor who could help you focus on the future. Choose someone familiar with the set-up in the country in which you plan to train in future.

Barrier No. 3: Fear of getting left behind

One reason you might avoid being in touch with friends and colleagues is that being in touch can trigger a fear of being left behind. But it's too easy to think of life as a race.

Box 11.2 Finding a quite different ethos

Joe is an emergency physician who left the UK after his foundation training for Australia. Joe planned for the trip to last a year. Once in Australia, however, he was asked if he would be willing to extend his contract which would mean delaying his return. At the time it was possible to train there in emergency medicine before applying for permanent residence—which made staying an attractive option. For Joe and many of his peers, they felt they needed a complete break from the UK. Looking back, and at other doctors' experiences of their stays, Joe thinks it helps to be self-motivated and fairly outgoing.

One of the changes that Joe and his peers had hoped for was to feel more valued. In the UK it had been commonplace to be upbraided for trivial misdemeanours—like drinking tea and coffee tacitly intended for patients. Of course, most doctors expect to be corrected—but the experience in Australia was of doctors' skills being more properly appreciated and rewarded with a better working week and better pay.

These differences seem to have prevailed to the present day. Knowing their rotas in advance means doctors can plan the rest of their lives. Joe still feels surprised that in Australia, rota requests by doctors are normally granted.

There are times when the emergency work is intense. Serious clinical situations occur regularly and can be traumatic for the team. But Joe's experience is that the quality of the teamwork makes such situations feel more manageable than they did in the UK.

As others progress to training programmes it can look like they're on course to net the most attractive posts. In reality opportunities open up at different times.

- Staying in touch with friends at home makes it more likely their experience will help you. There can be real advantages to hearing what they have to say.

- Remind yourself of the insights you have gained—not only about yourself but also about another healthcare system.

Summary

The role of the medical doctor is sufficiently similar around the world to make it feasible for doctors to work and travel. Yet the doctoring role is also sufficiently different around the world that the work can seem both exciting and challenging.

The completion of foundation training is a particular moment that lends itself for travel—although other times are also possible. Of course, not everybody wants to travel. But for those who do, the experience can give them valuable skills which are likely to strengthen subsequent job applications. Keeping in touch with colleagues back home and keeping track of the skills you acquire—as well as how you felt about your various experiences—will help when it comes to planning the next stage of your career.

References

1. **Brennan, N., Langdon, N., … & Humphries, N.** (2021). *Drivers of international migration of doctors to and from the United Kingdom.* **General Medical Council.** https://www.gmc-uk.org/-/media/documents/drivers-of-international-migration-research-final-report_pdf-88769526.pdf

2. **Parkhouse, J.** (1991). *Doctors' careers: aims and experiences of medical graduates.* Routledge.

3. **Silverton, R., & Freeth, D.** (2022). *The F3 phenomenon: Exploring a new norm and its implications.* Health Education England. https://www.hee.nhs.uk/sites/default/files/documents/F3_Phenomenon_Final.pdf

4. **Wilson, H.C., Abrams, S., & Simpkin Begin, A.** (2021). Drexit: understanding why junior doctors leave their training programs to train overseas: an observational study of UK physicians. *Health Sci Rep.* 4(4):e419. DOI: 10.1002/hsr2.419

5. **Sharma, A., Lambert, T.W., & Goldacre, M.J.** (2012). Why UK-trained doctors leave the UK: cross-sectional survey of doctors in New Zealand. *J R Soc Med.* 105(1):25–34. DOI 10.1258/jrsm.2011.110146

6. **Church, H., Agius, S., & Jenkins, L.** (2023). *The post-foundation training break ('F3'): evaluating its impact on postgraduate medical training. A report of independent research funded by the General Medical Council and Association for the Study of Medical Education.* https://www.gmc-uk.org/about/what-we-do-and-why/data-and-research/research-and-insight-archive/the-post-foundation-training-break-evaluating-its-impact-on-postgraduate-medical-training

7. **British Medical Association** (2024). Working abroad as a doctor—key considerations. https://www.bma.org.uk/advice-and-support/career-progression/working-abroad/work ing-abroad-as-a-doctor-key-considerations

8. **British Medical Association** (2023). Volunteering abroad as a doctor. https://www.bma. org.uk/advice-and-support/career-progression/working-abroad/volunteering-abroad-as- a-doctor

9. **General Medical Council** (n.d.). *Request a certificate to show your good standing with us.* https://www.gmc-uk.org/registration-and-licensing/managing-your-registration/certifica tes/request-a-certificate-of-good-standing-from-us

10. **General Medical Council** (n.d.). *Doctors working overseas.* https://www.gmc-uk.org/regis tration-and-licensing/employers-medical-schools-and-colleges/employing a doctor/doct ors-working-overseas

11. UK Foundation Programme (n.d.). F2 standalone. https://foundationprogramme.nhs.uk/ programmes/f2- stand-alone

12. **NHS Health Careers** (n.d.). *The idea of experiencing a novel healthcare system elsewhere in the world appealed to me.* https://www.healthcareers.nhs.uk/explore-roles/doctors/career-opportunities-doctors/real-life-story-f2-australia

13. **NHS England** (2023). *Certificate of readiness.* https://medical.hee.nhs.uk/medical-train ing-recruitment/medical-specialty-training/foundation-competencies/certificate-of-readiness

14. **General Medical Council** (n.d.). *Out of programme (OOP).* https://www.gmc-uk.org/ education/standards-guidance-and-curricula/guidance/out-of-programme

15. **NHS England** (n.d.). *Workforce, training and education.* https://www.hee.nhs.uk/our-work/dentists-training/delivering-greater-flexibility/out-programme

16. **Taber, B.J.** (2013). Time perspective and career decision-making difficulties in adults. *J Career Assess.* **21**(2):200–209. https://doi.org/10.1177/1069072712466722

Further reading

Junior Dr https://www.juniordr.com/advice-on-working-overseas/

Medic Footprints https://medicfootprints.org/the-benefits-of-working-abroad-for-your-career/

Médecins Sans Frontières (Medicine without Borders) https://msf.org.uk/

Medics Travel http://www.medicstravel.com/

NHS England—Global health partnerships https://www.hee.nhs.uk/our-work/global-eng agement

NHS England—Medical specialty recruitment https://medical.hee.nhs.uk/medical-training-recruitment/medical-specialty-training

NHS England—Working abroad https://heeoe.hee.nhs.uk/psw/support-services-available/ psw-support-providers/careers-support/working-abroad

NHS Scotland—Global Citizenship Programme. https://www.scottishglobalhealth.org/

NHS Wales—International Health Division https://phw.nhs.wales/services-and-teams/policy-and-international-health-who-collaborating-centre-on-investment-for-health-well-being/international-health-division/

Redr https://www.redr.org.uk/

UK-Med https://www.uk-med.org/

Voluntary Service Overseas (VSO) https://www.vsointernational.org/

Chapter 12

On being prepared

Medicine is a tough career. Our aim in this chapter is to build on doctors' awareness of the toll that the work and the work environment can take on their health and well-being. We start by discussing stress and burnout before going on to review doctors' mental health. It's natural to hope or believe these adversities won't happen to you personally. But we will discuss the statistical likelihood that you—or somebody with whom you work—might be affected. It can be hard to know what to do in either eventuality so we consider the ways in which doctors can seek help for themselves or their colleagues.

Stress

Many facets of our jobs have the potential to cause us harm. The list holds no surprises: excessive workload, insufficient control over our work and the imbalance that frequently occurs between the demands of work and its rewards.[1] But two individuals in the same job role may carry out their duties very differently, experiencing different levels of stress.[2]

The UK's work safety regulator, The Health and Safety Executive (HSE)[3] takes an unambiguous view, holding employers responsible for monitoring their employees' stress. The HSE define stress as 'the adverse reaction people have to excessive pressures or other types of demand placed on them'. Adverse reactions can take the form of burnout symptoms, physical symptoms, or the symptoms of mental illness. Employers are required not only to carry out risk assessments but also to act upon their findings. To do so they must actively manage six areas: the demands placed on employees, employees' degree of control, the support made available to employees, work relationships, work roles, and the process of changes.

The NHS and GMC monitor stress by surveying staff.[4,5] Most NHS staff surveys in recent years have found more than 40% of staff to suffer from stress-related symptoms. Around 40% of staff feel able to meet all the demands at work while only around 25% consider staffing levels to be sufficient to perform their jobs adequately. Moreover, it is known that around 40% of NHS staff sickness absence is likely to be related to stress.[6]

Burnout

Burnout isn't new. First described in 1974 by Freudenberger,[7] burnout has been extensively studied by Christina Maslach who found many types of emergency worker were prone to a syndrome comprising feelings of emotional exhaustion, emotional distancing from one's work and feelings of guilt and shame.[8] Extreme work demands, coupled with a personal drive to take on responsibility can lead employees to 'absorb' additional work over long periods. The worker juggles tasks, fearful of letting colleagues down, fearful of failure, or of being seen to be vulnerable.[9]

> ### Box 12.1 **ICD-11 Burnout**
>
> ◆ Feelings of energy depletion or exhaustion
>
> ◆ Increased mental distance from one's job, or feelings of negativism or cynicism related to one's job, and
>
> ◆ Reduced professional efficacy.
>
> Reprinted from *International Classification of Diseases*, Eleventh Revision (ICD-11). Geneva: World Health Organization; Copyright 2022. https://icd.who.int/en

The NHS Staff Survey finds worrying levels of both burnout and stress. More than a third of healthcare staff experience at least one symptom of burnout.[10,11] Frontline clinical staff are particularly vulnerable. Burnout is a particular occupational hazard for doctors, affecting 31% to 54%.[12] The GMC's 2022 National Training Survey showed 19% of trainees and 12% of trainers to be at high risk of burnout, while 63% of trainees and 52% of trainers were at moderate risk.[13]

Research has consistently shown that the underlying cause of burnout is not a lack of personal resilience because evidence indicates that the medical profession already selects for resilient people.[14] Instead, the primary causes of burnout are systemic and organizational, resulting from workloads and work cultures that place unachievable demands on their medical staff.

Because of the high prevalence of burnout, the World Health Organization (WHO) added the condition to the International Classification of Diseases (ICD-11) in 2019.[15] Although we often speak of 'symptoms' (Box 12.1), burnout is conceptualized by the WHO not as a disease but as an occupational phenomenon arising from chronic workplace stress that has not been successfully managed.

Mental health

While burnout may lead to mental ill-health, mental ill-health commonly occurs in its own right. Around one in four people in the general population in the UK are affected by mental health symptoms each year.[16] A systematic review and meta-analysis spanning 18 countries and taking in 17,500 doctors-in-training found the prevalence of clinical levels of depression to be 29%.[17] Around 24% of doctors experience clinical levels of anxiety while 4% to 16% experience post-traumatic symptoms.[18] Our appreciation of the effects of 'morally injurious events' is still developing. These are events that challenge people's deeply held moral values or beliefs.[19] We do know that occupational groups beyond the military experience post-traumatic stress symptoms following morally injurious events. For health staff we see associations between morally distressing events and the symptoms of burnout.[20]

Taking the symptoms of the various mental health disorders together, the proportion of doctors found to be affected varies between 17% and 52%.[12,21] Women, younger doctors, those working very long hours, and medical students are particularly vulnerable.

So what happens when doctors start to experience problems with their mental health? First, we know that doctors worry about making mistakes—about the quality of their advice to patients and about completing work tasks satisfactorily. Many feel unable to undertake additional responsibilities or work additional hours. A third of all doctors (and particular male and older doctors suffering mental ill-health) use alcohol or drugs to cope. Among those doctors with a lifetime diagnosis of a mental illness, the proportion using drugs or alcohol for coping may be as high as 62%.

A very significant concern when doctors are mentally unwell is, of course, suicide. In contrast to physical health, for which standardized mortality ratios (SMRs) for doctors are generally lower than for the general population, the SMR for suicide for doctors is higher than that of the general population, and especially high for female doctors.[22–24] Doctors' vulnerability may partly be explained by their greater knowledge and access to lethal suicide methods. But it may also be explained by doctors' *lesser* access to effective help.

What emerges is a picture of mentally ill doctors struggling to access help, working when unwell. In a series of in-depth interviews with 21 mentally ill doctors, Riley et al.[25] teased out the themes. The issues most important were the need to manage workloads and shift patterns in under-staffed contexts. When difficult clinical situations arose, experiencing difficulty accessing support from senior clinicians was a potent stressor. Inadequate physical spaces for de-briefing or rest was detrimental to the doctors. Over half had experienced abuse, bullying, felt devalued, intimidated, or humiliated. Some had experienced gender or race discrimination. When things went wrong clinically, doctors' experience was of being shamed and blamed rather than being supported.

Help-seeking

In our own practice we have been heartened to find that many doctors *do* now seek help from their GPs. GPs often have considerable experience with mental health and empathy for their distressed doctor-patients. GPs can encourage appropriate periods of sick leave, start treatment, and refer patients to more specialist services. If you wonder whether you yourself may be suffering from mental health symptoms, it's worth considering:

- What aspects of work, if any, may have contributed to your current state?
- Conversely, what aspects of work may be affected by your current state?
- Do you feel sad, tearful, empty, irritable, fearful, or suicidal?
- Are you worried by your use of alcohol or drugs?
- Have you managed to preserve time for a life beyond work?

What services exist?

- Practitioner Health was set up in 2008 to meet the needs of doctors, with mental or physical health problems, including addiction problems.
- DocHealth provides subsidized online therapy for doctors facing burnout, bullying, or harassment, relationship difficulties, stressors (such as receiving a complaint), and mental health difficulties.

- Many NHS trusts provide counselling as well as occupational health services. Burnout is mostly commonly managed by modifying people's working hours (including on-call duties). But burnout can also be helped by learning mindfulness skills and developing coping skills. In one systematic review, team-based cognitive behavioural therapy (CBT) was more effective for burnout than individual interventions[26] but it's uncommon for UK health providers to be able to offer interventions of this kind.

- Clinical and educational supervisors can often signpost doctors to support services like the Professional Support Units provided by the LETBs (local education training boards). These can provide both career support and support for disabilities including dyslexia, autism, or ADHD.

If you feel concerned about confidentiality (or its limits), ask the practitioner to explain how confidentiality works in practice.

Resilience

Resilience is 'the ability to adapt well in the face of significant stress and adversity, to recover from difficulties and to potentially gain strength from them'.[27] Those scoring lowest on resilience scales are more likely to experience burnout symptoms.[28–30] Such findings must, however, be considered alongside the research discussed earlier showing the primary drivers of burnout to be systemic rather than individual. Even if the root cause of burnout is not any lack of personal resilience, we may, to some extent, still be able to safeguard our well-being by increasing our resilience. So how might we do this?

Firstly certain personal qualities may contribute to resilience—attributes like extraversion, self-esteem, and optimism. It's also possible to learn to become both more optimistic and more resilient with the help of CBT or in the case of resilience, developing mindfulness skills has been shown to be helpful.[31–33] Resilience is now seen as sufficiently important to be included in the medical school professionalism curriculum[34] and is promoted by NHS organizations.[35]

Resilience (and its lack) is an attribute that whole teams can possess. Team resilience is 'the capacity of a team to withstand and recover from challenges, pressure, or stressors and to bounce back'.[36] That *team* resilience is starting to be studied is refreshing as doing so shifts the responsibility from the individual to the team as a whole. One quantitative study demonstrated associations between team resilience, the quality of leadership, the quality of the teamwork and the team's efficacy.[37]

In a review of qualitative studies of organizational resilience (with 12 healthcare organizations), Barasa et al.[38] found resilient organizations to be distinct in that:

- Resources were made more available and/or are used more strategically
- The organizations collaborated differently with other organizations
- The flow of information was more effective
- The organizations used multiple ways to achieve their goals
- Control was 'distributed' rather than 'centralized'
- Their leaders were visible, available, and communicated a clear vision

- The cultures of the organizations promoted learning
- The staff were sufficiently numerous, supported, motivated, and resourceful

The limited evidence suggests that it is high-quality leadership that makes the difference. It is worth noticing resilience when it occurs in the teams and organizations in which you work—and what seems to maintain any resilience.

Well-being

Well-being can be defined as 'a state of happiness and contentment, with low levels of distress, overall good physical and mental health and outlook, or good quality of life'.[39] One model gaining traction on account of the under-pinning evidence-base is the *PERMA* model.[40] Individuals are more likely to achieve well-being if their needs are met in terms of:

- **P**ositive emotions—such as hope, curiosity, pride, and compassion
- **E**ngagement—being able to become absorbed in activities, 'flow' (as discussed in Chapter 2 of this book) is an example of what is meant by engagement
- **R**elationships—experiencing the support of others, a sense of social connectedness, friendship, being positively regarded
- **M**eaning—experiencing a sense of purpose and belonging
- **A**ccomplishment—accomplishing things that are personally important

With well-being in mind, the GMC undertook an independent review of doctors' working lives. The resulting report, *Caring for Doctors, Caring for Patients*[41] concluded that doctors' well-being depended on three pre-requisites: Autonomy, Belonging, and Competence (ABC). Unpacking the elements of ABC (Box 12.2), it's possible to notice similarities with those of PERMA.

Soon after *Caring for Doctors, Caring for Patients* was published, the pandemic occurred. Its impact may in part account for these important principles not achieving the prominence they deserved. With deteriorating working conditions cited in the recent pay dispute between the government and medical staff, it is fair to say that doctors are not seeing many of the systemic changes called for. One can only hope that this work is still pending.

Perfectionism and shame

Many doctors are perfectionists, being driven to perform as flawlessly as is humanly possible. This is not surprising as doctors' selection is based upon near-perfect exam results. But perfectionism can also be a health hazard. Personality traits of neuroticism when coupled with introversion are associated with mental ill-health.[12] Perfectionism is associated with burnout symptoms[42,43] and can precipitate depression when setbacks occur.[44]

How might this work? It seems that perfectionists with particularly high fear of mistakes are less willing to talk to others when their performance slips.[45] It is likely that one of the most upsetting of emotions, shame, may be implicated. Brené Brown defines shame as 'the intensely painful feeling or experience of believing that we are

Box 12.2 **Caring for doctors, caring for patients**

Autonomy

- Doctors (and other clinicians) need to have a voice in organizations' decision-making.[53]
- Learning rather than blame should characterize the culture of organizations.
- Facilities and rotas should conform to certain minimum standards.
- Fatigue should inform shift patterns, swaps, and realistic forecasting.

Belonging

- Experiencing mutual caring, respect, and being valued is important within organizations.
- A sense of belonging can result from working within effective multidisciplinary teams.
- Compassionate leadership also fosters a sense of belonging.

Competence

- Workload reviews enable competencies to develop and high-quality care to be delivered.
- Managers and supervisors should meet doctors' basic need for supervision and education.
- Medical educators (and indirectly, the GMC) can enhance students' well-being by providing confidential services and flexible placements.
- Well-being, compassion, and team-working should form part of the curriculum.
- Personal development plans should be encouraged.
- Formative types of assessment should complement traditional 'pass-fail' exams.

Data from West, M., & Coia, D. (2019). Caring for doctors, caring for patients. General Medical Council. https://www.gmc-uk.org/-/media/documents/caring-for-doctors-caring-for-patients_pdf-80706341.pdf

flawed and therefore unworthy of love and belonging'.[46] Yet we know that a sense of belonging is important for our well-being. Brown considers that just as shame arises within social relationships, its harmful effects could be ameliorated through social means: being able to speak about the subject with those whom we respect.

Organizations can perpetuate or mitigate shame. A multi-site study by management scholar Amy Edmonson attests to this. US intensive care staff were significantly more likely to follow the guidelines for the self-reporting of drug errors if the unit's manager was independently rated as supportive and accessible.[47] Such managers took a non-blaming approach, conveying an understanding of the universality of human error.

The findings suggest that the selection and training of leaders could be one way to reduce the harmful effects of shame in organizations and teams.

Supporting staff by providing Schwartz Rounds may also help. Kenneth Schwartz, a Bostonian healthcare lawyer noticed something that might seem obvious during his own cancer care: the difference it makes to patients when staff show compassion. Schwartz set up a centre for compassionate healthcare[48] which has since promoted Schwartz Rounds. UK Schwartz Rounds are hour-long facilitated events that enable multidisciplinary staff to talk together about their experience of delivering care when challenges have occurred. It can be difficult to achieve good attendance but those who do attend report improvements in their well-being.[49]

Having reviewed some of the ways in which we can be better prepared, we now want to consider how this might work in practice (Box 12.3).

Box 12.3 Burning out in good company

An ambitious plastic surgery trainee, Sandra, came to recognize that she was suffering from burnout. Sandra's experience of stress developed when studying for her FRCS. Not only was she struggling to gain sufficient experience operating, but her team was led by a series of locum consultants due to sickness. The trust was struggling to recover from COVID-19. Various changes affected the theatres. Sandra was willing to work hard at night and hoped this would be rewarded. Where possible, she opted into rota gaps. The nights were busy but often did not provide the right kind of training experience.

Sandra's well-being deteriorated after she made a mistake when on-call. Though on the face of it, she was well-supported, Sandra felt devastated and broke down in her interview with the serious incident investigator. Sandra's educational supervisor suggested Sandra join a mentoring scheme for women. Sandra was paired with a mentor right away.

Sandra's mentor suggested Sandra complete a burnout questionnaire. It became apparent that Sandra was not only exhausted, but she thought she was not doing a good-enough job. This was burnout. The jolt motivated Sandra to make some changes. She knew she had become isolated from her family and friends and wasn't as fit as she wanted to be. So Sandra joined a gym and booked sessions with a personal trainer. Next she joined a knitting circle at work (where she was the only doctor). But the knitting circle punched above its weight, leading to a breakthrough: the other knitters helped Sandra realize that filling rota gaps was counterproductive for her. Somehow, she'd got into the mindset of being hyper-aware of the cost of locums, that information often being disseminated by management. Sandra decided to hand back 'ownership' of the problem to those who perhaps should have taken greater ownership all along.

Several years on, Sandra has passed her exams and was granted an out-of-programme leave to work with an organization that is training her to work close to conflict zones. Recognizing the signs of burnout was an important step on the journey. Sandra realizes the strong link between being highly driven and burnout. She did not have to change her long-term plan—just her approach to seeking support and making adjustments.

We have considered burnout and mental ill-health at one end of a spectrum, and wellness and resilience at the other. We have looked at some of our personal vulnerabilities and some of the organizational factors that can help or impede us in our endeavours. This chapter would not be complete without looking—albeit briefly—at some of the specific situations that have the power to negatively impact on well-being.

Bullying, harassment, and discrimination

Bullying at work is unwanted behaviour from a person or group that is offensive, intimidating, malicious, insulting, or a misuse of power. Bullying becomes harassment if it is related to a characteristic protected by the 2010 Equality Act: age, gender reassignment, marriage or civil partnership, pregnancy or maternity leave, disability, race, nationality, ethnicity or national origin, religion or belief, sexual orientation, or sex.[50] Two in five doctors experience bullying or harassment.

Direct discrimination involves people being unfavourably treated because they (or a person with whom they are associated) has a protected characteristic.[51] Indirect discrimination occurs if a rule or practice means that people with a protected characteristic are treated less favourably. Not allowing staff to cover their heads, for example, indirectly discriminates against those who do so for religious or cultural reasons.

If you believe you may have experienced bullying, harassment, or discrimination:

- Note what happened, when and where it took place, who was involved or may have witnessed what happened.

- Talk to any witnesses, and to those who have a duty of care towards you. Consider escalating the matter to a senior or human resources.

- If a member, consult with the BMA.

- With support, consider what would restore your well-being. A supported meeting or mediation meeting may help.

- An investigation may determine if the organization's policies have been breached.

Complaints and investigations

Feeling that your work is being scrutinized or that you are to blame when something has gone wrong is particularly distressing. Receiving a complaint is associated with an increased risk of depression and anxiety. Ongoing complaints are associated with a heightened risk of the doctor considering self-harm or even suicide. Practitioner Health looked at the cohort of doctor-patients who had used their services.[52] Ten per cent of the whole cohort had had the experience of some level of GMC involvement. For the group of doctors who had died from any cause, 52% had experienced GMC involvement. It is safest to conclude that referral to the GMC may be a risk factor for doctors in terms of suicide.

If you experience heightened distress in response to things going wrong:

- Seek support from seniors and professional supporters as well as your family and friends.

- Talk to your medical indemnifier, the BMA, or other legal supporter.

- Seek the support of your GP, a counsellor, therapist, or Practitioner Health—as a matter of urgency if you experience suicidal thoughts or feelings.
- Treat yourself with the same compassion you would a close friend. This is the principle of self-compassion. Psychologist Kristin Neff provides a range of self-compassion suggestions at self-compassion.org (see Further reading section).

Raising concerns

The GMC's ethical standards *Good Medical Practice*[53] states that doctors have a duty to raise concerns if patient safety, dignity, or comfort is at risk. The few studies that have focussed on raising concerns in health settings suggest that organizations are able to respond and learn when concerns are raised, but their ability to do so depends on good organizational leadership. Unfortunately, organizations can sometimes 'resist' learning leaving the person who raised the concerns in a state of emotional distress.[54,55]

- Talk to your supervisor or manager. Sometimes it is necessary to escalate concerns to a person at a more senior level—even to the chief executive officer. Before reaching out to an external body, discuss the issue with a confidential and very trustworthy advisor.
- Consider whether it may be safer to raise concerns as a *group* of concerned doctors. Your ability to do so may depend upon the circumstances of the case.
- Study your organization's 'whistle-blowing' or 'raising concerns' policy before acting.
- Seek the confidential advice of your medical indemnifier and the BMA.
- If the situation does not resolve, you are likely to need ongoing advice and emotional support.
- Keep a comprehensive record of your concerns, dates, communications, and the advice you receive.

We have discussed situations that constitute the greatest risks to doctors' well-being. But we want to highlight that very difficult situations can be (and often are) turned around. Working as a doctor is usually a deeply rewarding vocation.

We will end the chapter by briefly considering job satisfaction—but we first return to a topic already touched on: compassion. Increasingly we hear about compassion in healthcare and in health leadership.[56] There is accumulating evidence for the importance of delivering compassionate healthcare, not only for the sake of the patients but also for staff well-being. It is important to acknowledge that an important driver has been those situations in which compassion was found to be sadly lacking. In the UK, the Mid Staffordshire context is the best-known example in which hundreds of patients received grossly sub-optimal care culminating in many excess deaths.

Compassionate healthcare

Compassion is defined as an emotional response to another's pain or suffering which involves an authentic desire to help and goes beyond feeling empathy. Compassion is specifically about taking effective action to lessen a person's or people's suffering.[57] Cochrane et al. describe the practices carried out in those hospitals and community settings in the US and Canada which exemplify compassionate care.[58] The key features include:

- Leadership styles which are communication-rich and compassion-laden
- Recruitment and induction focus on compassion
- New staff are trained in the required organizational values and skills
- There is a whole-person and pro-active approach. Patient needs are anticipated rather than waiting for the patient to make a request
- The organizations overtly value diversity and difference

It is conceivable that in order to be able to effectively deliver compassionate healthcare, practitioners are best advised to *also* practice self-compassion. Paradoxically, to do so, staff may need to resist the urge to overwork.[59] It may be easier to achieve this delicate balance when working as part of resilient team. Conversations with a trusted supervisor, a mentor, or through participating in facilitated conversations like Schwartz Rounds are also likely to help.

Job satisfaction

It's important to remind ourselves that there is such a thing as job satisfaction—defined as the 'pleasurable or positive emotional state resulting from the appraisal of one's job or job experiences'.[60] Notwithstanding some of the difficult issues we have discussed, many doctors *do* experience a deep sense of job satisfaction. So despite all the stresses it revealed, the 2022 NHS Staff Survey suggested that 53% of staff looked forward to going to work and 67% felt enthusiastic about their jobs.

Being consciously aware of job satisfaction when it occurs is likely to enhance staff well-being.[41] Journalling with a particular focus on the positive moments in a so-called gratitude log has now come into the mainstream. Downloadable templates are available from Positive Psychology.com, listed at the end of this chapter.

Summary

We have tackled some of the tough topics in the knowledge that the levels of stress, burnout, and mental ill-health run at high levels in the medical profession. Never before has it seemed so necessary for doctors to be forewarned about the problems they might encounter in their work. We hope too that these topics, which are now beginning to be included in the medical curriculum, can be openly discussed throughout your career, leading to a more supportive culture across the profession as a whole.

References

1. **Michie, S.** (2002). Causes and management of stress at work. *Occup Environ Med.* **59**(1):67–72. https://doi.org/10.1136/oem.59.1.67

2. **Harris, C., Daniels, K., & Briner, R.B.** (2004). How do work stress and coping work? Toward a fundamental theoretical reappraisal. *Br J Guid Couns.* **32**(2):223–234. https://doi.org/10.1080/03069880410001692256

3. **Health and Safety Executive** (n.d.). Stress and mental health at work. https://www.hse.gov.uk/stress

4. **NHS** (2024). NHS staff survey. https://www.nhsstaffsurveys.com

5. **General Medical Council** (n.d.). *The state of medical education and practice in the UK: workforce report 2023.* https://www.gmc-uk.org/about/what-we-do-and-why/data-and-research/the-state-of-medical-education-and-practice-in-the-uk/workforce-report

6. **Rimmer, A.** (2018). Staff stress levels reflect rising pressure on NHS, says NHS leaders. *BMJ.* **360.** DOI: 10.1136/bmj.k1074

7. **Freudenberger, H.J.** (1974). Staff burn-out. *J Soc Issues.* **30**(1):159–165. https://doi.org/10.1111/j.1540-4560.1974.tb00706.x

8. **Kinman, G., & Teoh, K.** (2017). They took off their uniform when they got home, but couldn't remove the armour. *The Psychologist.* **30**:58–61.

9. **Ekstedt, M., & Fagerberg, I.** (2005). Lived experiences of the time preceding burnout. *J Adv Nurs.* **49**(1):59–67. https://doi.org/10.1111/j.1365-2648.2004.03264.x

10. **Taylor, C., Graham, J., … & Ramirez, A.J.** (2005). Changes in mental health of UK hospital consultants since the mid-1990s. *Lancet.* **366**(9487):742–744. https://doi.org/10.1016/S0140-6736(05)67178-4

11. **Matthew-King, A.** (2018). *Revealed: the rising tide of GP burnout as NHS cuts support.* Pulse.

12. **Imo, U.O.** (2017). Burnout and psychiatric morbidity among doctors in the UK: a systematic literature review of prevalence and associated factors. *BJPsych Bull.* **41**(4):197–204. DOI: 10.1192/pb.bp.116.054247

13. **General Medical Council** (2024). National training survey reports. https://www.gmc-uk.org/about/what-we-do-and-why/data-and-research/national-training-surveys-reports

14. **Shanafelt, T., Trockel, M., … & Bohman, B.** (2019). Building a program on well-being: key design considerations to meet the unique needs of each organization. *Acad Med.* **94**(2):156–161.

15. **World Health Organization.** (2019, May 28). Burn-out an 'occupational phenomenon': International Classification of Diseases. https://www.who.int/news/item/28-05-2019-burn-out-an-occupational-phenomenon-international-classification-of-diseases

16. **McManus, S., Meltzer, … & Jenkins, R.** (2009). *Adult psychiatric morbidity in England: Results of a household survey.* Health and Social Care Information Centre.

17. **Mata, D.A., Ramos, M.A., … & Sen, S.** (2015). Prevalence of depression and depressive symptoms among resident physicians: a systematic review and meta-analysis. *JAMA.* **314**(22):2373–2383. DOI:10.1001/jama.2015.15845

18. **Harvey, S.B., Epstein, R.M., … & Henderson, M.** (2021). Mental illness and suicide among physicians. *Lancet.* **398**(10303):920–930. https://doi.org/10.1016/S0140-6736(21)01596-8

19. **Norman, S.B., Nichter, B., … & Pietrzak, R.H.** (2022). Moral injury among US combat veterans with and without PTSD and depression. *J Psychiatr Res.* **154.** 190–197. https://doi.org/10.1016/j.jpsychires.2022.07.033

20. **Lamiani, G., Borghi, L., & Argentero, P.** (2017). When healthcare professionals cannot do the right thing: a systematic review of moral distress and its correlates. *J Health Psychol.* **22**(1):51–67. https://doi.org/10.1177/1359105315595120

21. **Bhugra, D., Sauerteig, S.O., . . . & Ventriglio, A.** (2019). A descriptive study of mental health and wellbeing of doctors and medical students in the UK. *Int Rev Psychiatr.* **31**(7-8):563–568. DOI:10.1080/09540261.2019.1648621

22. **Hawton, K., Clements, A., . . . & Deeks, J.J.** (2001). Suicide in doctors: a study of risk according to gender, seniority and specialty in medical practitioners in England and Wales, 1979–1995. *J Epidemiol Commun Health.* **55**(5):296–300. https://doi.org/10.1136/jech.55.5.296

23. **Schernhammer, E.S., & Colditz, G.A.** (2004). Suicide rates among physicians: a quantitative and gender assessment (meta-analysis). *Am J Psychiatry.* **161**(12):2295–2302. https://doi.org/10.1176/appi.ajp.161.12.2295

24. **Dutheil, F., Aubert, C., . . . & Navel, V.** (2019). Suicide among physicians and health-care workers: a systematic review and meta-analysis. *PloS One.* **14**(12):e0226361. https://doi.org/10.1371/journal.pone.0226361

25. **Riley, R., Buszewicz, M., . . . & Chew-Graham, C.** (2021). Sources of work-related psychological distress experienced by UK-wide foundation and junior doctors: a qualitative study. *BMJ Open.* **11**(6):e043521. DOI: 10.1136/bmjopen-2020-043521

26. **Panagioti, M., Panagopoulou, E., . . . & Esmail, A.** (2017). Controlled interventions to reduce burnout in physicians: a systematic review and meta-analysis. *JAMA Int Med.* **177**(2):195–205. DOI:10.1001/jamainternmed.2016.7674

27. **McCain, R.S., McKinley, N., . . . & Kirk, S.J.** (2018). A study of the relationship between resilience, burnout and coping strategies in doctors. *Postgrad Med J.* **94**(1107):43–47. DOI: 10.1136/postgradmedj-2016-134683.

28. **Olson, K., Kemper, K.J., & Mahan, J.D.** (2015). What factors promote resilience and protect against burnout in first-year pediatric and medicine-pediatric residents? *J Evid-Based Complementary Altern Med.* **20**(3):192–198. https://doi: 10.1177/2156587214568894

29. **McKinley, N., McCain, R.S., . . . & Kirk, S.J.** (2020). Resilience, burnout and coping mechanisms in UK doctors: a cross-sectional study. *BMJ Open.* **10**(1):e031765. DOI: 10.1136/bmjopen-2019-031765

30. **Di Trani M., Mariani R., . . . Frigo M.G.** (2021). From resilience to burnout in healthcare workers during the COVID-19 emergency: the role of the ability to tolerate uncertainty. *Front Psychol.* **16**(12):646435. DOI: 10.3389/fpsyg.2021.646435

31. **Robertson, I.T., Cooper, C. L., Sarkar, M., & Curran, T.** (2015). Resilience training in the workplace from 2003 to 2014: a systematic review. *J Occup Organiz Psychol.* **88**(3):533–562. https://doi.org/10.1111/joop.12120

32. **Joyce, S., Shand, F., . . . & Harvey, S.B.** (2018). Road to resilience: a systematic review and meta-analysis of resilience training programmes and interventions. *BMJ Open.* **8**(6):e017858. https://doi.org/10.1136/bmjopen-2017-017858

33. **Kunzler, A.M., Helmreich, I., . . . & Lieb, K.** (2020). Psychological interventions to foster resilience in healthcare professionals. *Cochrane Database Syst Rev.* **7**. https://doi.org/10.1002/14651858.CD012527.pub2

34. **Gishen, F., Lynch, S., Gill, D., Jawad, S., & Peters, D.** (2018). Medical student resilience: a symposium approach. *Clin Teach.* **15**(5):425–427.

35. **Alliger, G.M., Cerasoli, C.P., . . . Vessey, W.B.** (2015). Team resilience: how teams flourish under pressure. *Organ Dyn.* **44**(3):176–184. https://doi.org/10.1016/j.orgdyn.2015.05.003

36. **Barratt, C.** (2018). Developing resilience: the role of nurses, healthcare teams and organisations. *Nurs Stand.* **33**(7):43–49. DOI: 10.7748/ns.2018.e11231

37. **Vera, M., Rodríguez-Sánchez, A.M. & Salanova, M.** (2017). May the force be with you: looking for resources that build team resilience. *J Workplace Behav Health.* **32**(2):119–138. https://doi.org/10.1080/15555240.2017.1329629

38. **Barasa, E., Mbau, R., & Gilson, L.** (2018). What is resilience and how can it be nurtured? A systematic review of empirical literature on organizational resilience. *Int J Health Policy Manag.* **7**(6):491. DOI: 10.15171/ijhpm.2018.06

39. **American Psychological Association** (2024). APA dictionary of psychology. https://dictionary.apa.org/well-being

40. **Seligman, M.** (2011). *Flourish: a new understanding of happiness and wellbeing—and how to achieve them.* Nicholas Brealey Publishing.

41. **West, M., & Coia, D.** (2019). *Caring for doctors, caring for patients.* General Medical Council. https://www.gmc-uk.org/-/media/documents/caring-for-doctors-caring-for-patients_pdf-80706341.pdf

42. **McManus, I.C., Keeling, A., & Paice, E.** (2004). Stress, burnout and doctors' attitudes to work are determined by personality and learning style: a twelve year longitudinal study of UK medical graduates. *BMC Med.* **2**:1–12. DOI: 10.1186/1741-7015-2-29

43. **Martin, S.R., Fortier, M.A., . . . & Kain, Z. N.** (2022). Perfectionism as a predictor of physician burnout. *BMC Health Serv Res.* **22**(1):1425. DOI: 10.1186/s12913-022-08785-7.

44. **Flett G.L. & Hewitt P.L.** (2002) *Perfectionism theory, research, and treatment.* American Psychiatric Association.

45. **Frost, R.O., & DiBartolo, P.M.** (2002). Perfectionism, anxiety, and obsessive-compulsive disorder. In: Flett, G.L. & Hewitt, P.L., eds. *Perfectionism theory, research, and treatment.* American Psychological Association; 341–371. https://doi.org/10.1037/10458-014

46. **Brown, B.** (2013). *Shame versus guilt.* https://brenebrown.com/articles/2013/01/15/shame-v-guilt

47. **Edmondson, A.C.** (1996). Learning from mistakes is easier said than done: Group and organizational influences on the detection and correction of human error. *J Appl Behav Sci.* **32**(1):5–28. DOI: 10.1177/0021886304263849

48. **The Schwartz Center** (2024). Putting compassion at the heart of healthcare. https://www.theschwartzcenter.org

49. **Maben, J., Taylor, C., . . . & Foot, C.** (2018). A realist informed mixed-methods evaluation of Schwartz Center Rounds® in England. *HSDR.* **6**(37):1–260. https://doi.org/10.3310/hsdr06370

50. **BMA** (2018). *Bullying and harassment: how to address it and create a supportive and inclusive culture.* https://www.bma.org.uk/media/1100/bma-bullying-and-harassment-policy-report-oct-2019.pdf

51. **BMA** (2022). Discrimination advice for doctors. https://www.bma.org.uk/advice-and-support/equality-and-diversity-guidance/discrimination-guidance/discrimination-advice-for-doctors

52. **Gerada, C.** (2018). Doctors, suicide and mental illness. *BJPsych Bull.* **42**(4):165–168. DOI: 10.1192/bjb.2018.11

53. **General Medical Council.** *Good medical practice.* https://www.gmc-uk.org/professional-standards/professional-standards-for-doctors/good-medical-practice

54. **Lim, C.R., Zhang, M.W., . . . & Ho, R.C.** (2021). The consequences of whistle-blowing: an integrative review. *J Patient Saf.* **17**(6):e497–e502. DOI: 10.1097/PTS.0000000000000396

55. **Augustine, L.G.** (2022). Whistleblowing in healthcare for patient safety: an integrative literature review. *Int J Hum Res Stud.* **12**(1):1531–1531. https://doi.org/10.5296/ijhrs.v12i1.19477

56. **The King's Fund** (2022). *What is compassionate leadership?* https://www.kingsfund.org.uk/publications/what-is-compassionate-leadership

57. **Trzeciak, S., Mazzarelli, A., & Booker, C.** (2019). *Compassionomics: the revolutionary scientific evidence that caring makes a difference.* Studer Group.

58. **Cochrane, B.S., Ritchie, D., … & Nelson, B.** (2019, May). A culture of compassion: How timeless principles of kindness and empathy become powerful tools for confronting today's most pressing healthcare challenges. *Healthc Manag Forum.* **32**(3):120–127.

59. **McKee, A., & Wiens, K.** (2017). Prevent burnout by making compassion a habit. *Harvard Business Review.*

60. **Locke, E.A.** (1976). The nature and causes of job satisfaction. In: Dunnette, M.D., ed. *Handbook of industrial and organizational psychology.* Rand McNally; 1297–1343.

Further reading

Brown, B. (2015). *Daring greatly: how the courage to be vulnerable transforms the way we live, love, parent, and lead.* Penguin Books.

Doherty, M., Johnson, M., & Buckley, C. (2021). Supporting autistic doctors in primary care: challenging the myths and misconceptions. *Br J Gen Pract.* **71**(708):294.

Harris, R. (2022). *The happiness trap: stop struggling, start living*, 2nd edition. Robinson.

Hennessey, G. (2016). *The little mindfulness workbook.* Hodder & Stoughton.

Kross, E. (2022). *Chatter: the voice in our head.* Vermilion.

Williams, M., & Penman, D. (2011). *Mindfulness: a practical guide to finding peace in a frantic world.* Hachette.

Further information

Autistic Doctors International https://autisticdoctorsinternational.com
Canopi (Wales) https://canopi.nhs.wales/about-us/
DocHealth https://www.dochealth.org.uk
Practitioner Health https://www.practitionerhealth.nhs.uk
Positive Psychology https://positivepsychology.com/gratitude-journal
The Samaritans https://samaritans.org/
Self-compassion https://self-compassion.org
The Workforce Specialist Service (Scotland) https://wellbeinghub.scot/the-workforce-specialist-service-wss

Chapter 13

A whole career

Career planning isn't limited to choosing your specialty; it's an iterative process that starts before you go to medical school and continues throughout your working life, up to and including retirement. In other words, career planning is best seen as a process rather than an event. Our needs change both gradually and in abrupt ways which can take us by surprise. The healthcare context too is always changing and presenting challenges. All this means it's never too late to start career planning, and for those who did so before, there's every reason to re-kindle the habit from time to time.

We first want to consider career success and job satisfaction and we review the impact of individual and organizational factors on whether or not you experience your work as rewarding. Next we look at what you can do to gain the support you need throughout your career. We give special consideration to mentoring, to seizing opportunities, and to reviewing your career along the way. We make no apologies for adhering to the same career planning stages that we outlined in Chapter 1—albeit with one or two adaptations—and we offer a couple of new exercises as well.

Career success and career satisfaction

Most of us intuitively know what career success should look and feel like yet might find it hard to pin it down precisely. In the research literature, career success has been defined in objectively measurable ways: earnings, position, and status. More recently it has come to be accepted that our subjective career satisfaction is equally important: Did we accomplish what we had hoped to accomplish? How do we feel looking back on our career journey? How do we see our future career options? All these things make up career success, defined as 'the positive psychological and work-related outcomes accumulated as a result of one's work experiences'.[1] Subjective career satisfaction differs from job satisfaction which we discussed in Chapter 12 in that it is the summation of positive work experiences over a whole career. Both are important.

Career success, satisfaction, and me

If you carried out some of the self-knowledge exercises in Chapter 2, you may have found yourself attributing some of the events to the kind of person that you are—in other words, to your personality. Personality is 'the enduring configuration of characteristics and behaviour that comprises an individual's unique adjustment to life—traits, interests, drives, values, self-concept, abilities, and emotional patterns'.[2] Five personality traits are particularly well recognized—'the Big Five'—having been robustly validated in personality research. These are extraversion/introversion, neuroticism, openness to experience, agreeableness, and conscientiousness. Three of these, extraversion, conscientiousness, and openness to experience are found to be associated with career success.[1,3] Extraversion and conscientiousness require little explanation. Openness to experience is descriptively named: it is about being broadminded and willing to try new things.

A further individual difference important for career satisfaction is Proactive Personality. Though not one of the 'Big Five', Proactive Personality is favoured by those recruiters (outside the medical world) who regularly use personality questionnaires. People high in proactivity 'take initiative to influence their surroundings'.[4] The association between Proactive Personality and job performance is greater than for the Big Five personality traits.[5,6] It's also worth noting that Proactive Personality may overlap with some of the other individual characteristics discussed earlier in this book—characteristics like 'grit' and 'growth mindset'. All have at their core the ability to persevere.

Another characteristic with a bearing on career satisfaction is optimism. To be optimistic, is of course, to expect good things to happen. The disposition is associated with generally favourable moods and greater motivation than is its polar opposite, pessimism. Optimism is also associated with lower cardiovascular morbidity and all-causes mortality,[7] perhaps because of differences in people's coping styles. Optimists tend to use problem-orientated ways of coping for the more controllable types of problem and are less likely than pessimists to cope by withdrawing from situations, denying them, or wishing things were different.[8]

A growing literature demonstrates the relationships between such characteristics as grit and optimism on the one hand, and well-being, satisfaction, performance, and perseverance on the other. Loftus et al. summarized the findings of 52 studies for US surgeons at the time of the pandemic.[9] We summarize the review's take-home messages in Box 13.1.

Fortunately, it's possible for those who were not born optimistic to learn to be more so. Martin Seligman, one of the originators of positive psychology as a subdiscipline, devotes several chapters of his book *Learned Optimism*[10] to coaching the reader through several simple steps based upon cognitive behavioural therapy (CBT) techniques.

Box 13.1 **Advice at times of COVID-19**

- ◆ Maintain optimal levels of positivity.
- ◆ It can be helpful to recall what has gone well each day.
- ◆ Negative events can be seen positively as opportunities to learn.
- ◆ Pursue major challenges that match [your] personal skills.
- ◆ Engage in deliberate practice to improve [your] personal skills.
- ◆ Persist in hard work over time, valuing effort over talent.
- ◆ Pursue higher meaning and purpose in work and life.

Reprinted from *The American Journal of Surgery*, 220, 1, Loftus TJ et al., 'Performance advantages for grit and optimism', pp. 10-18, Copyright 2020, with permission from Elsevier. https://doi.org/10.1016/j.amjsurg.2020.01.057

We might wonder if optimism could have a downside. As a clinician you will know to guard against excessive optimism when you have to deliver news about a potentially devastating prognosis. In other circumstances too—particularly when the stakes are high, or when other people's futures are at stake—engaging with *some* level of pessimism can allow you to assess situations more accurately. So there is a balance to be struck—a balance which Seligman calls, 'flexible optimism'.

Putting the 'we' into our careers

Career satisfaction and career success are not only about you. When discussing resilience in Chapter 12, we highlighted the potential importance of team and organizational resilience. We might wonder what effects team and organizational factors may have on individuals' career satisfaction. The volume of research is modest but lends support to the importance of factors that go beyond the individual. In particular, our career satisfaction is greater if we have been able to access more training. We are also influenced by the nature of the work we carry out[11] and the level of support we receive.[12] It is important not only to be rewarded but also to perceive a level of fairness in the way resources are allocated.[13,14] Not surprisingly then, individual and external factors are both important.

It is tempting to assume that equivalent levels of support are available throughout the NHS but you may well know from experience that there is actually considerable variation. An implication of this is that when you are able to exercise greater choice (upon completing your training for example), you should try to assess the availability of support that is likely to exist before making a final decision as to which job to take. At every stage it is worth looking out for opportunities for training and support.

Mentoring

Mentoring is a process in which an experienced, highly regarded, empathic person guides another, usually younger, person in their learning and/or professional development. The mentor achieves this simply through listening and talking confidentially with the mentee.[15] Mentoring support is increasingly available through both employing organizations and professional organizations (like deaneries and royal colleges). Research generally suggests that mentees find the process satisfying but a couple of studies stand out as they go a little further.

In a study of the effects of mentoring over two years,[16] the authors controlled for factors that would be expected to affect mentees' career success—the extent of the mentees' training, Proactive Personality, and the extent of mentees' networks. While mentoring did not influence mentees' pay by the end of the study period, the mentoring did influence whether mentees' had been promoted and their expectations about their future career advancement.

In another interesting study, mentoring was provided under the auspices of an Australian health and medical research gender equity initiative. Most mentees improved in their knowledge of diversity and inclusion and most felt better able to conduct a 'difficult workplace conversation' should the need arise. Many saw more general improvements in how they communicated with colleagues and were better placed to identify promotion and grant opportunities[17].

Opportunities

Serendipity is important for romantic storylines and also lies behind some of the significant medical discoveries. The story of the discovery of penicillin is an example, resting on Alexander Fleming seizing on a chance event in his laboratory. We might wonder if an opportunity were to occur in our lives, would we recognize it as such? And how can we be better prepared to make the most of chance events when they do come our way?

An interesting study addressed this question. Legrand and her team studied hundreds of French managers, asking them to recount any chance events that had occurred over their careers. They also asked them to describe any effects of the events that they perceived.[18] Many had experienced chance events—meeting a particular person, an organizational restructuring, redundancy, or experiencing a personal loss, as well as many other types of event. Surprisingly, both positive and negative chance events were more likely to be followed by career effects that were perceived positively. Those managers describing positive career effects were more likely to score highly on measures of 'protean career orientation' and 'employability'. Protean career orientation is a measure of taking personal responsibility for one's career goals. Employability is a subjective measure of career success. So what the study seems to suggest is that the effect of chance events may be part of a wider pattern about the impact of one's personal outlook. Of course what this study cannot tell us is whether we can *learn* to open our eyes to hidden opportunities in events as they occur—but that is a possibility, particularly given that we can learn to become more optimistic.

Responding to opportunities

In reviewing your own career, a good starting point is to consider chance events and how you have responded to them so far:

◆ One approach is to revisit your career lifeline (see Chapter 2). For each segment of the lifeline, you might wonder if a positive or negative chance event had occurred. If so, with what effects? You may be able to work out why the event had those particular effects—if it had to do with your mindset at the time, what was happening in your life, or perhaps the influence of role models.

◆ Were there occasions when you could have taken an opportunity but didn't? If so, imagine turning back the clock and taking the alternate path (as in the film, *Sliding Doors*). Where might the opportunity have led? What might you be doing now? We are not suggesting you should 'beat yourself up' about not having taken an opportunity but that should you want to, you can learn to be better prepared for a future opportunity that might occur. Or you could even search out an opportunity.

◆ It's worth wondering how an opportunity might present itself—through an advert or email, or might somebody mention something? The word 'opportunity' can be over-used or mis-applied to jobs. To distinguish, you might consider, 'Where could this lead?' 'How interesting (or otherwise) could this turn out to be?' or 'How does this fit (or not fit) with my own interests, skills and needs?'

Reviewing your career

We have promised to adhere to the structure described in Part 1 of this book. The structure is essentially to separate the processes of attending to self-knowledge (making explicit your interests, skills, and needs) and exploring the 'out there' opportunities.

In reviewing your career, you'll be more interested to update your self-knowledge by reviewing the job roles you've had and your developing interests. By yourself or with a mentor (or other trusted person), the following prompts may help:

- Can you recall what motivated you to enter the field you now work in?

- What did you most hope to achieve?

- To what degree have you achieved what you had hoped to achieve (or are on a path to achieving these things)?

- How relevant do your earlier goals feel today? Have your goals changed? If so, is this a consequence of developing new interests or discovering new talents? Alternatively might any change in your goals relate to external factors, e.g. organizational change, new research, progress, or technological change?

- What gives you greatest satisfaction? Re-visiting the Experience Log (Chapter 2) could help you answer this question.

- What's your theory as to why you experience the elements of your role the way you do?

- How well are you matched to the elements that make up your job role?

- How do others regard your work and accomplishments? If you have a 360-degree appraisal, what do others see as your strengths? Do their perceptions of your relative weaknesses accord with your own? Alternatively, you could ask one or more trusted colleagues for their impressions: in what contexts do they see you functioning at your best and most contentedly?

- How does your personality influence the way you work? Consider your level of extraversion or introversion (preference for working with others or alone), proactivity, your tendency to worry (or not) and how conscientious you are.

- Do you want to change anything about your approach to work? Many people want to be more confident, more proactive, or to have better boundaries. These are topics typically discussed with mentors and coaches.

- What might you like to accomplish next?

- Are you satisfied with your current job role?

- How do you see the future of your specialty? Are there particular skills you think you think you'll need to acquire in future? If so, how can you acquire these skills?

- What new opportunities do you perceive—in terms of specific activity, patient group, setting, training, status, or pay?

- How do you see your role models or peers progressing?
- What about your work–life balance? How effectively do you control your workload?

Can appraisal help with career planning?

In the UK, annual appraisal forms part of the revalidation cycle. Perhaps for this reason, appraisal can lean more towards being summative than being developmental. *Good Medical Practice* encourages reflection that aims to improve your professional practice rather than your career satisfaction. But good appraisers often strive to make appraisals meaningful in subjective career terms. Since we know that self-knowledge can be made explicit in many different ways, it is conceivable that insights could arise as you prepare for an appraisal, or during the appraisal itself.

What's possible?

Where previously a job was a job for life, we now hear of doctors moving from one post to another, their career taking all sorts of interesting directions. We have encountered doctors who implemented changes to their working lives to great positive effect. They include:

- Doctors who studied for an additional qualification, funding their own studies, or negotiating the funding with their employer. It's easier to be funded for leadership or management courses—or to acquire skills for services that your organization needs.

- Doctors who became medical educators.

- Doctors who became clinical academics. When there are shortages of clinical academics, it may be more possible to move into research at a stage a little later than might otherwise be possible.[19] The Clinical Academic Training and Careers Hub, (CATCH)[20] provides information about academic pathways.

- Doctors, frustrated by working in serial locum posts, who have later been successfully appointed to substantive posts as consultants or GPs.

- Doctors who have taken up sessions or moved entirely into the private sector allowing greater autonomy, the ability to deliver care differently, or meet family caring needs.

- Doctors who reduced their hours to take on a side project—that is, an activity alongside their 'day job'. We have heard of side projects in complementary medicine, psychotherapy, comedy, growing flowers, yoga, and entrepreneurship. A side project can sometimes be a staging post for a later career change.

- Doctors typically retire younger than do the general population.[21] Those in shortage specialties may be particularly well-placed to negotiate and could consider working fewer hours and developing a side project (or developing their non-work interests) in preparation for later retirement.

As with many of our case studies, the case studies that follow in Boxes 13.2, 13.3 and 13.4 are inspired by doctors we know. You may also know inspiring role models like them—or can look out for role models. Medic Footprints, whose website is listed at the end of the chapter, is also an excellent source of inspiration.

> ## Box 13.2 **A portfolio career in general practice**
>
> Vanessa is a mid-career GP and GP trainer. Vanessa chose not to become a partner. Doing so might have constrained her from developing her interests to her satisfaction. Resisting that particular duty has allowed Vanessa to keep her career fresh.
>
> When the practice appointed a physician associate (PA), the need to appoint a PA supervisor also arose. At the time, Vanessa knew little about the PA role but as a 'can-do' person, she quickly unearthed the information she needed and took on the PA supervisor role. Several related opportunities opened up in quick succession, all of which went to Vanessa: educational supervisor for the PAs, developing a CPD programme for the PAs and as the local PA workforce expanded, there was a need for somebody to support the PA supervisors.
>
> As Vanessa gained experience in medical education, she had no trouble in being appointed to a medical school tutor role, and thence to a role as lead tutor. Vanessa finds delivering the school's communication skills training one of her most satisfying work duties. Another source of job satisfaction is her work for the Professional Support Unit, supporting doctors at risk of not passing their SCA exam and doctors returning from maternity leave.
>
> Vanessa was recently asked to apply for a role providing women's health clinics at a prison in her area. Opportunities like this keep coming along—making it necessary to look critically at all her roles together—at the time and energy each requires. Could an older project be handed on to a successor to make space for something new?
>
> Reviewing her career, Vanessa reflected on the autonomy she has. Developing and maintaining a large network of colleagues while also being embedded in a good GP practice gives Vanessa a real sense of belonging. She also recognizes the importance for her of 'giving back' in the support she provides to her younger colleagues.

Possible barriers to career review

Barrier No. 1: Loyalty to colleagues

Many doctors are highly conscientious—to the extent of working even when sick. Contemplating asking for a change to your job plan—let alone leaving a service—can feel disloyal to trusting colleagues. But consider that:

- If you come to experience burnout, your colleagues would then be affected. Finding ways to increase your career satisfaction may reduce your risk of burnout, ultimately benefitting everybody.

- As a role model for others, attending to your own long term career satisfaction may increase other people's chances of doing the same.

- Your colleagues wouldn't want you to sacrifice yourself. You may wish to check if this is the case by asking them. But hopefully you'll be pleased by their responses.

Box 13.3 **Developing artistically**

From childhood, Paula loved to draw, spending much of her spare time creating pictures. As a teenager, she won an art competition. At high school, Paula reached the point of having to choose between studying advanced maths and art. Her heart said art – but being very academic, Paula aimed for a career in medical science. After her first degree (in philosophy, psychology, and physiology) and graduate training in pharmacology, Paula pursued a D.Phil at Oxford University. Paula's lab books told an interesting story, covered as they were with illustrations. They highlighted the strength of the pull Paula still felt towards the world of art, even while she was training scientifically.

Paula went on to qualify as a clinical doctor, and completed an academic foundation programme. She then began her specialty training. But while there were aspects of the job she loved, she felt worn down by her working hours, frustrated by her location, and worried about the limited scope for innovation. Paula took a bold step: she arranged to break from her medical training and immerse herself in art. Though she had not been to art school, Paula was able to compile a portfolio from the products of her many years of sketching, printing, and photography. These efforts paid off: Paula was accepted onto a prestigious master's course in illustration, at the Cambridge School of Art.

On the course, Paula began to thrive, relishing the artistic freedom afforded by her new situation – in particular, the opportunity to develop her own individual style. All this was very different to Paula's experience of her medical training. Unlikely as it might seem, there were some interesting cross-overs between Paula's two professional lives. The attention to detail that had been necessary to develop as a doctor now served Paula well in training as an illustrator, and Paula's scientific background proved invaluable in helping her explore the technical side of printmaking.

Paula continued to teach medical students, at the University of Cambridge, while working on various book projects. In early 2025, with the award of a Harvard Radcliffe fellowship to support her in writing and illustrating a children's book about death, Paula's creativity was gaining global attention. Tragically, Paula died several months before she could start on the next chapter of her extraordinary career.

Barrier No. 2: Lack of confidence

You may have an exciting idea only to be paralysed by a sense of embarrassment for having dared to think you could do it. Imposter syndrome can make an appearance at any stage. In such a situation:

◆ Take courage from the talented individuals who have openly discussed their own experience of imposter syndrome.

◆ Recall the Duning-Kruger effect (discussed in Chapter 8) which shows that we can be quite poor judges of our abilities. Highly skilled people may under-rate their ability.

◆ Recall Duckworth's concept of 'Grit' (discussed in Chapter 4) and that *effort may be more valuable than talent.*

Box 13.4 **A portfolio career in psychiatry**

Karl qualified in Germany and went on to train in Child and Adolescent Psychiatry (CAMH) in the UK. But now he works with adults rather than children. He is also head of the School of Psychiatry for his deanery.

Karl was a highly regarded CAMH psychiatrist who began to feel unfulfilled. It seemed that the demand was increasing while the funding was being squeezed. The constant need to divide his time between his various clinical responsibilities rankled as he needed to focus on the patients with severe eating disorders. In contrast, Karl found greater job satisfaction in his educational role, supervising trainees.

A colleague and friend, Lydia, had been a superb Training Programme Director (TPD) for the region's CAMH training. Karl sometimes took on delegated tasks to support Lydia, doing so primarily for his own interest. He was keen to provide a learning environment that was different from the traditional training he himself had experienced. Lydia, knowing that she planned to move on, encouraged Karl to study for a PG Cert in Medical Education. Initially he wondered if another course would be a chore but he actually found the training stimulating. Importantly, having done the course, Karl was in a strong position to successfully apply for the TPD role when the opportunity occurred. Once appointed, he found working with the trainees made him more optimistic about the future of CAMH.

As a full-time CAMH consultant Karl seemed always to be on-call. The crunch came when a family holiday to visit Karl's parents in Germany had to be cancelled due to a consultant rota problem.

Next, a chance event occurred: a consultant in the adult eating disorders service resigned. Karl, it was suggested, should apply. The idea seemed a stretch—could a CAMH eating disorder consultant really treat adults? Karl talked the question over with friends. It was Lydia who pointed out that Karl had more than sufficient skill to do the role exceptionally well. Karl had no wish to give up his TPD role but how could he continue while working with adult patients? A second chance event occurred (sometimes a series of such events really can happen). The head of school announced their retirement. Once again Karl was in a position to apply and was duly appointed.

Nowadays Karl is always busy but his roles no longer conflict with each other. He was able to bring his CAMH expertise to his work with adults. As if this variety was not enough, Karl now also has a 'side project' that allows him to keep his CAMH skills alive.

So what is Karl's secret? He thinks that having a curious mind has been a factor as well as his tendency to ask himself, 'How can I make this work?' He poses this question not just to himself but also to friends. So noticing and creating opportunities and having supportive friends at work are also important.

◆ It is well known to CBT practitioners that when anxious, we tend to make catastrophic predictions. To reduce the impact, ask, 'What would I advise a friend in this situation?', 'What's the worst thing that could happen?', and 'What's the best thing that could happen?'

Barrier No. 3: The time not being right

Sometimes despite needing and wanting a change, the timing is just not right. Too much else may be happening in your life.

◆ If you have to put your ideas on hold in order to attend to more pressing concerns, don't give up on your ideas altogether. You might set a date to reconsider your ideas. The same idea may still be valid later—or perhaps a different (and maybe even better) opportunity will later present itself.

Summary

We included this chapter because we wanted to emphasize that career planning is not just something you do in your foundation years or in the early years of specialty training. That was just the beginning—and the reality is that throughout your working life there are so many choices, they would be overwhelming without a structured approach to career planning (Figure 13.1). If there's a lot going on at work or in your personal life, it can be tempting not to plan. For this reason, it's helpful to gain support wherever possible. We hope that this book gives you a sense of support and that our case studies are an inspiration.

Our parting wish is for you to benefit from that special combination of ingredients: luck, optimism, support, and grit.

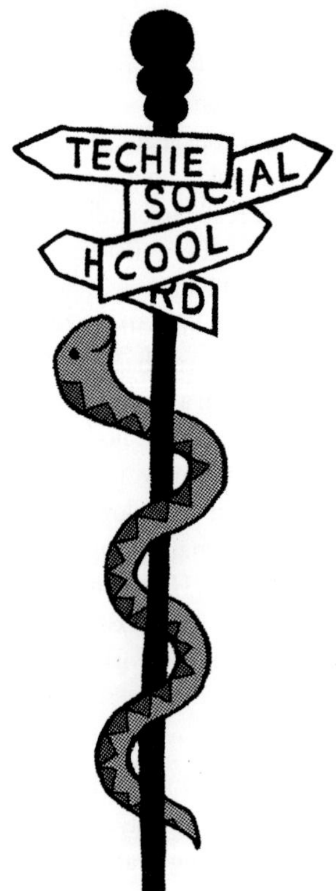

Figure 13.1 It can be hard to see the opportunity when faced with multiple paths
A choice of interesting and appealing paths to go down.

References

1. **Seibert, S.E., & Kraimer, M.L.** (2001). The five-factor model of personality and career success. *J Vocat Behav.* **58**(1):1–21. https://doi.org/10.1006/jvbe.2000.1757

2. **American Psychological Association** (2024). APA dictionary of psychology. https://dictionary.apa.org/personality

3. **Lounsbury, J.W., Loveland, J.M., … & Hamrick, F. L.** (2003). An investigation of personality traits in relation to career satisfaction. *J Career Assess.* **11**(3):287–307. https://doi.org/10.1177/1069072703254501

4. **Bateman, T.S., & Crant, J.M.** (1993). The proactive component of organizational behavior: a measure and correlates. *J Organ Behav.* **14**(2):103–118.

5. **Fuller Jr, B., & Marler, L.E.** (2009). Change driven by nature: a meta-analytic review of the proactive personality literature. *J Vocat Behav.* **75**(3):329–345. https://doi.org/10.1016/j.jvb.2009.05.008

6. **Spitzmuller, M., Sin, H.-P., … & Fatimah, S.** (2015). Investigating the uniqueness and usefulness of proactive personality in organizational research: a meta-analytic review. *Hum Perform.* **28**(4):351–379. https://doi.org/10.1080/08959285.2015.1021041

7. **Craig, H., Freak-Poli, R., … & Gasevic, D.** (2021). The association of optimism and pessimism and all-cause mortality: a systematic review. *Pers Individ Differ.* **177**:110788.

8. **Nes, L.S., & Segerstrom, S.C.** (2006). Dispositional optimism and coping: a meta-analytic review. *Pers Soc Psychol Rev.* **10**(3):235–251. 10.1207/s15327957pspr1003_3

9. **Loftus, T.J., Filiberto, A.C., … & Upchurch Jr, G.R.** (2020). Performance advantages for grit and optimism. *Am J Surg.* **220**(1):10–18. https://doi.org/10.1016/j.amjsurg.2020.01.057

10. **Seligman, M. E. P.** (2018). *Learned optimism: how to change your mind and your life.* John Murray Press.

11. **Tharenou, P., & Conroy, D.** (1994). Men and women managers' advancement: personal or situational determinants? *Appl Psychol.* **43**(1):5–31. https://doi.org/10.1111/j.1464-0597.1994.tb00807.x

12. **Türe, A., & Akkoç, İ.** (2020). The mediating role of social support in the effect of perceived organizational support and psychological empowerment on career satisfaction in nurses. *Perspect Psychiatr Care.* **56**(4). DOI:10.1111/ppc.12562

13. **Rhoades, L., & Eisenberger, R.** (2002). Perceived organizational support: a review of the literature. *J Appl Psychol.* **87**(4):698–714. https://doi.org/10.1037/0021-9010.87.4.698

14. **Renee Barnett, B., & Bradley, L.** (2007). The impact of organisational support for career development on career satisfaction. *Career Dev Int.* **12**(7):617–636. DOI:10.1108/13620430710834396

15. **Standing Committee on Postgraduate Medical and Dental Education** (1998). *Supporting doctors and dentists at work: an enquiry into mentoring.* SCOPME.

16. **Singh, R., Ragins, B.R., & Tharenou, P.** (2009). What matters most? The relative role of mentoring and career capital in career success. *J Vocat Behav.* **75**(1):56–67. https://doi.org/10.1016/j.jvb.2009.03.003

17. **Vassallo, A., Walker, K., … & Joshi, R.** (2021). Do mentoring programmes influence women's careers in the health and medical research sector? A mixed-methods evaluation of Australia's Franklin Women Mentoring Programme. *BMJ Open.* **11**(10):e052560. DOI: 10.1136/bmjopen-2021-052560

18. **Legrand, C., Naschberger, C., … & Bozionelos, N.** (2023). Chance events in managers' careers: positive and negative events, their expected and unexpected outcomes. *Eur Manag Rev.* **20**(3):461–476. https://doi.org/10.1111/emre.12546

19. **British Medical Association** (2018). Mid-career entry to academic medicine. https://www.bma.org.uk/media/1376/bma-mid-career-entrants-to-medical-academia-july-2018.pdf

20. **Catch.** Welcome to the clinical academic training and careers hub. https://www.catch.ac.uk

21. **Smith, F., Goldacre, M.J., & Lambert, T.W.** (2018). Retirement ages of senior UK doctors: national surveys of the medical graduates of 1974 and 1977. *BMJ Open.* **8**(6). DOI: 10.1136/ bmjopen-2018-022475

Further information

Medic Footprints—https://medicfootprints.org

Index

For the benefit of digital users, indexed terms that span two pages (e.g., 52–53) may, on occasion, appear on only one of those pages.

Boxes are indicated by an italic *b* following the page number.